CW00524621

A VETERINARY
MATERIA MEDICA
and
CLINICAL REPERTORY

Other works by G. Macleod

THE TREATMENT OF HORSES BY HOMOEOPATHY
THE TREATMENT OF CATTLE BY HOMOEOPATHY
THE HOMOEOPATHIC TREATMENT OF DOGS
CATS: HOMOEOPATHIC REMEDIES

A
VETERINARY
MATERIA MEDICA

AND
CLINICAL REPERTORY
WITH A MATERIA MEDICA
OF THE NOSODES

BY

G. MACLEOD
M.R.C.V.S., D.V.S.M.
ASSOCIATE OF THE FACULTY OF HOMOEOPATHY

VETERINARY CONSULTANT TO MESSRS A. NELSON & CO
MANUFACTURERS OF HOMOEOPATHIC MEDICINES

VETERINARY CONSULTANT TO THE BRITISH
HOMOEOPATHIC ASSOCIATION

VETERINARY CONSULTANT TO THE
HOMOEOPATHIC DEVELOPMENT FOUNDATION

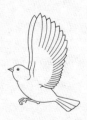

THE C. W. DANIEL COMPANY LTD
SAFFRON WALDEN

First published in Great Britain by
The C. W. Daniel Company Ltd
1 Church Path, Saffron Walden, Essex, England

© G. Macleod 1983
Reprinted 1989

SBN 85207 154 X

Set in 10 on 11 Plantin by the White Crescent Press Ltd, Luton
and printed by Hillman Printers of Frome, Somerset.

CONTENTS

PREFACE

This materia medica of the commoner remedies used in veterinary practice has been compiled in the hope that it will assist the owners of animals to determine which remedy is likely to be the most effective when treating the simpler conditions with which he or she may be confronted. It is not intended to be a complete study of the remedies mentioned, for which a standard materia medica should be consulted. As much care as possible has been taken to eliminate all subjective symptoms, and the more obvious objective signs have been concentrated on. The remedies mentioned in the repertory of the commoner conditions have relevance mainly to the text of the main work and it must be stressed that they are by no means exhaustive as reference to a more complete repertory will show.

The author hopes that this materia medica will be used in conjunction with the other works which have been published on horses and cattle, as it should make for easier understanding. In the chapter on bowel nosodes, I acknowledge the pamphlet by the late Dr John Paterson.

Finally, I wish to express my sincere thanks to Mrs Diana Killick for her patience in typing the manuscript so carefully and expeditiously and for coping with some rather unusual nomenclature. Without her assistance the work might still be in long hand.

G. Macleod
Lindfield, March 1983

Abies Canadensis

Hemlock Spruce. *N.O.* Coniferae. The buds of the young plant and the fresh bark provide the material for the Ø.

This plant has an affinity for mucous membranes generally and that of the stomach in particular, producing a catarrhal gastritis. There is a tendency to prostration and fever, and also to over-eat.

Alimentary System. Mouth generally dry. After eating abdominal rumblings are heard. Impairment of liver function occurs leading to flatulence and deficient flow of bile. The appetite is increased and hunger may be ravenous. Constipation is usually present.

Renal System. Urination is frequent, even during the night, the urine being straw-coloured.

Female Genital System. An action on the uterus occurs which leads to a tendency to displacement. This may lead to straining with possible prolapse.

Respiratory System. Laboured breathing.

Cardiac System. Heart's action is laboured with an increased action.

Extremities. Muscular twitchings are seen. General prostration.

Skin. This is cold and clammy and the animal may show shivering because of a reduction in surface temperature.

USES

It is mainly to be considered as a remedy for alimentary conditions of small animals, particularly gastritis with catarrhal vomiting, accompanied by a torpid liver function. Animals which benefit from its use will probably show the characteristic cold skin and shivering along with excessive craving for food.

Abies Nigra

Black Spruce.   *N.O.* Coniferae.   The tree secretes a gum which is the source of the Ø.

This is a long-acting remedy producing mainly gastric symptoms, especially in older subjects. Conditions are worse after eating which brings on abdominal discomfort. The animal becomes restless towards nightfall.

Alimentary System.   Before mid-day there is loss of appetite but this returns towards evening, but any food eaten brings about uneasiness. Constipation is present.

Respiratory System.   Inspiration is difficult, especially in the recumbant position. A laryngeal cough is common.

Cardiac System.   Chest symptoms are accompanied by a heavy and slow heart's action.

Extremities and Muscular System.   Pain is evinced by pressure over sacral region. The animal may cry out because of limb pains.

USES

In the older dog showing stomach upset it could be a useful remedy. One should look for the characteristic signs of aggravation after eating, accompanied by loss of appetite in the morning with hunger at night. The gastric condition will probably be accompanied by vomiting, and while this is not a commonly used remedy in veterinary practice it undoubtedly has a place among remedies acting on the stomach. It may also prove of value in the treatment of certain types of heart weakness in the older dog.

Abrotanum

Southernwood.   *N.O.* Compositae.   The Ø is made from the stems and fresh leaves.

This plant shows an affinity with the muscular system and connective tissue producing a state of marasmus or wasting of the lower limbs and leading to a weakness in which the subject is unable to stand.

Alimentary System.   The Appetite remains good, but wasting becomes progressive. In the dog, cat and pig there may be vomiting of undigested material. Distension of abdomen occurs while constipation and diarrhoea may alternate. In young subjects there frequently appears an umbilical discharge or oozing which in the new-born may take the form of pure blood. Symptoms are generally worse at night.

Muscular System.   Weakness of neck and back muscle is prominent along with lameness and stiffness of joints. The head may appear heavy. Excessive emaciation of the lower limbs is a strong guiding symptom, the wasting developing from below upwards. Pain develops over the sacral region, symptoms being relieved by movement.

Skin. Eruptions occur together with a flabbiness of tissue. There may be loss of hair, while the skin assumes a bluish colour underneath.

USES

This is a useful remedy in marasmatic conditions, especially of older subjects. It has been used successfully in venous oozing from the umbilicus in the new-born animal, where loss of blood threatens to become serious. As a vermicide, used in low potency its main action is against ascaris worms. Post-influenzal weakness in the horse should benefit, while its action on the musculo-skeletal system suggests its use in rheumatism of small joints. In this connection diarrhoea frequently alternates with a rheumatic tendency. In the dog and cat it should be remembered as one of the remedies which might help in eruptive skin conditions with bluish discolouration and a tendency to alopecia.

Absinthum

Common Wormwood. *N.O.* Compositae. The Ø is prepared from the flowers and fresh young leaves of the plant.

The picture of this remedy is characterised by epileptiform seizures consequent on cerebral irritation and preceded by chorea and nervous tremors. This nervous excitement produces vertigo with a tendency to fall backwards.

Head. Spasmodic facial twitching occurs with fixation of jaws. There is unequal dilation of pupils of the eye while the head is kept low. The tongue is thickened and protrudes from the mouth.

Alimentary System. A bloated abdomen accompanies a flatulent colic, while there is a loss of appetite, and in the dog, cat and pig vomiting occurs. Swelling and tenderness develop over the liver region.

Renal System. There is excessive urination, the odour of the urine being strong and ammoniacal with a deep orange-yellow colour.

Respiratory System. There is a reflex cough dependent on liver dysfunction.

Cardiac System. Irregular heart action with a thumping sound which produces a full pulse.

Extremities. Symptoms of paralysis may appear.

USES

The nervous sequelae of canine distemper may call for this remedy, when it should be employed in fairly high potency. It could also be of use in the early development of tetanus. Cerebro-cortical necrosis of cattle and sheep should benefit as an adjunct to thiamine therapy, helping to prevent relapses. The abdominal symptoms suggest its use in flatulent colic of the horse, other symptoms being equal. Liver dysfunction leading to the appearance of orange-yellow urine may also benefit. Epileptiform attacks in the dog, whatever the cause, should improve under its use.

Aceticum Acidum

Glacial Acetic Acid. Characteristic of this remedy is anaemia associated with dropsical states accompanying a picture of severe wasting and debility with a tendency to haemorrhages. A strong guiding symptom is polyuria, the urine being pale and accompanied by intense thirst.

Head. Nasal catarrh with occasional epistaxis. Pupils of eyes become dilated.

Alimentary System. Salivation accompanies thirst except in fevered states when thirst is absent. Gastric involvement produces vomiting in the dog, cat and pig, often with haemorrhage from the bowels. Abdominal tympany is present along with ascites and diarrhoea, the latter often alternating with constipation.

Respiratory System. A croupous cough may arise which is worse on inhalation. Dyspnoea is eased by the animal assuming sternal recumbency.

Extremities. There is general emaciation and in the larger animals oedema of the lower limbs occurs.

Skin. Feverish conditions produce an erythematous state, the skin being burning hot.

Renal System. Large quantities of pale urine are voided. The urine contains phosphates and great thirst and debility are accompanying features.

Female Genital System. Mammary glands become enlarged and full, the milk being thin and bluish. Bleeding from the uterus is a common feature, especially post-partum.

USES

The remedy has been used successfully in diabetes in the dog, where emaciation and dropsy have developed. The haemorrhagic tendency of the remedy should be noted. It could have a place in the treatment of lymphangitis in the horse and in certain forms of mastitis in cattle, other symptoms agreeing. Putrid fevers may call for its use when accompanied by intense thirst.

Aconitum Napellus

Monkshood. *N.O.* Ranunculaceae. The Ø is derived from the whole plant along with the root, and is made when the plant begins to flower. All parts contain aconitine, the active alkaloid. There is an affinity with serous membranes and muscular tissues, leading to functional disturbances. Involvement is sudden and there is a generalised tension.

Eyes. Become red and inflamed with swollen lids producing lachrymation, fear of bright light and evidence of pain or discomfort. Pupils are dilated.

Ears. The external ear becomes red, hot and painful to the touch.

Respiratory System. Coryza with sneezing attempts may lead to epistaxis, the blood being bright red. Dyspnoea occurs with dry cough after exposure to cold dry winds. Bleeding from lungs may take place. Signs of pain or uneasiness may be seen on inspiration. Choking attacks are common. Pneumonia may supervene with heat of body, thirst, dry cough and nervous excitability.

Circulatory System. The pulse is full, hard and tense dependent on an increased heart beat. In fine-skinned animals the tension in the blood-vessels may make the carotid arteries visible as thick cords.

Alimentary System. Thirst is intense, possibly arising from swollen dry throat. The abdomen is sensitive to the touch. This may be due to the frequency with which the peritoneum becomes inflamed which in turn may arise from enteritis accompanied by diarrhoea or dysentery.

Extremities. Joints become swollen and hot. Synovitis is frequently encountered, especially in the larger joints.

Skin. Erythema develops with miliary eruptions and a fine red rash which becomes worse at night. The skin is hot and swollen-looking.

Renal System. There is a tendency to suppression. The urine is hot and assumes a reddish colour.

Female Genital System. There may be bleeding from uterus post-partum and sometimes yellowish discharge. Mammary glands may be swollen and secrete milk.

USES

This remedy should be used in the early stages of all feverish states. Where there is sudden appearance of symptoms which may show aggravation when any extreme of temperature occurs. Predisposing factors which may produce a drug picture calling for Aconitum include shock, operation, exposure to cold winds or dry heat. It is of use in puerperal fever quickly arising with peritoneal complications, and has given excellent results in tension of blood-vessels with epistaxis and other bleeding, e.g. in race-horses. It will be helpful in milk fever as an adjunct to calcium therapy. Animals which exhibit fear, e.g. of crowds or strange places will benefit.

Actaea Spicata

Baneberry.   *N.O.* Ranunculaceae.   The Ø is prepared from the root. The affinity of this plant is with the connective tissue of muscles and small joints, leading to painful conditions which are worse from touch and movement.
   Alimentary System.   Increased salivation. Tenderness over the epigastric region with vomiting in the dog and cat.
   Respiratory System.   Shortness of breath on exposure to cold air.
   Renal System.   Tendency to urinary calculi. White sediment in urine.
   Extremities.   Painful swelling of small joints, e.g. carpus and tarsus. Joint swellings may appear after prolonged walking or running.

USES
Should be considered in small joint rheumatism of old dogs. A useful remedy for joint swellings appearing after exercise, e.g. in the greyhound.

Adonis Vernalis

Pheasant's Eye.   *N.O.* Ranunculaceae.   An infusion or tincture of the whole plant is used. The action of the plant is mainly on the circulatory system, producing various pathological conditions affecting the action of the heart.
   Alimentary System.   Examination of the mouth reveals a shiny tongue and gums. The tongue may appear yellow and there is usually great hunger.
   Circulatory System.   Regurgitation of blood through the mitral valve accompanies disturbance of the aortic valve with inflammation of the main artery. Both peri- and endocarditis may be present. Marked venous engorgement occurs leading to irregular heart action. The pulse is rapid and irregular as a consequence.
   Renal System.   Urine is albuminous, scanty and shows an oily pellicle.
   Extremities.   Because of faulty heart action, oedema of various parts appears, notably ascites in the dog and lower limb swellings in the larger animal. Cattle may show brisket oedema.

USES

This is one of many valuable heart remedies, useful in canine practice
especially. Should be considered in cases of cardiac dropsy, in Bright's
Disease, and in asthmatic conditions of old subjects with coughing and
suffocative breathing. Post-influenzal weakness in the horse will benefit, the remedy helping to prevent myocardial weakness. Fog-fever in
cattle with lung oedema should also benefit. In the treatment of Valvular Disease it should be given in low potency, e.g. lx or a few drops of
Ø in water.

Aesculus Glabra

N.O. Sapindaceae.   The whole ripe fruit is employed in the preparation of the Ø. The main action of the plant is on the rectum, sacrum and
lower extremities with a tendency towards paresis of various parts.
   Head.   Vertigo, producing a staggering gait. Consciousness may
be lost. Eyesight may be lost with eyes assuming a fixed look.
   Alimentary System.   Vomiting occurs in small animals. Tympany of abdomen is a fairly constant feature. Severe constipation. Dark
red anal tumours are typical.
   Extremities.   A wry-neck condition may appear. Weakness of
lower back produces lameness with a tendency to collapse and paresis.
Tendon contraction of limbs is frequently encountered, spasms and
trembling of muscles.

USES

It could prove a useful remedy in the treatment of anal adenoma in the
dog, preventing deterioration and alleviating discomfort. Paretic conditions of cattle with muscular contractions, including wry-neck, should
benefit. It is one of the remedies to be remembered as an adjunct to
mineral therapy in the treatment of milk-fever and hypomagnesaemia.

Aesculus Hippocastanum

Horse Chestnut.   *N.O.* Sapindaceaea.   The Ø is prepared from the
entire fruit, including the capsule. The main affinity is with the lower
bowel producing a state of venous congestion. There is a general slowing down of the digestive and circulatory systems, the liver and portal
action particularly becoming sluggish.
   Eyes.   Lachrymation with engorged blood-vessels. Eyes have a
swollen look.
   Alimentary System.   Salivation with coated tongue. The throat

is markedly affected producing a follicular pharyngitis with distension of veins. Tenderness is evident over the hepatic and epigastric regions associated with liver congestion and jaundice. Rectal prolapse may occur with stools large, hard and dry, and showing a swollen congested mucosa. Vomiting and retching occurs in the dog.

Renal System.   Frequency of urination with passage of dark scanty urine which may contain a mucous sediment.

Circulatory System.   Heart action is full and heavy. Pulsation may be felt in usual places, e.g. a jugular pulse.

Respiratory System.   Coughing, with mucus, especially in the morning. Cough may be dependent on hepatic disorders and is usually catarrhal. Swelling of turbinate bones occurs with congestion and softening.

Extremities.   Weakness over sacral region which may give out on walking. Synovitis of tarsal joints may be seen, more especially the left. Pain over hamstrings.

USES

This is a useful remedy in liver conditions associated with venous congestion affecting the general circulation. Hock swellings in the horse, e.g. Spavin (Bog) may be relieved. As the name implies chest conditions of horses come within its sphere of action when dependent on congestions associated with coughing, made worse by inhalation of cold dry air. It should be considered in weakness affecting the sacro-iliac region especially those appearing after short exercising. Throat inflammations showing the typical engorgement of local blood-vessels suggest its use. Also similar condition affecting the eyes. Frequent yawning in the horse is sometimes a pointer to its use in digestive upsets.

Aethusa Cynapium

Fool's Parsley.   *N.O.* Umbelliferae.   Tincture of the whole flowering plant is used in preparation.

The brain and nervous system are affected by this plant, symptoms being associated also with disturbances of the gastro-intestinal tract. Signs of mental anguish appear which in the young animal may be connected with dentition and an inability to digest the mother's milk. Symptoms may appear suddenly.

Head.   Vertigo, increased by movement. Head shaking with restlessness and an anxious expression.

Eyes.   Photophobia and swelling of meibomian glands. Pupils dilated and eyes drawn downwards. Ophthalmia may occur together with swelling of eyelids.

Alimentary System.   Aphthous lesions may appear in a dry mouth with a pustular eruption in the throat. There is marked intolerance of milk which is regurgitated in curd form. In the dog, cat and pig frothy white vomition occurs shortly after eating while in all animals signs of abdominal colic appear. The stool is undigested, greenish and thin, but occasionally constipation occurs. Young animals may show chorea-like symptoms accompanied by coldness.

Respiratory System. A hoarse respiration accompanies an anxious expression. Coughing frequently occurs.

Lymphatic System. The lymph glands of the neck and axillae become swollen.

Circulatory System. Violent palpitation of the heart with rapid, small pulse.

Skin. Becomes cold and clammy. Itching eruptions occur around joints, which are worse from heat. Small cutaneous haemorrhages develop along with oedema of underlying tissues.

Renal System. Frequent passage of urine containing a sediment which is sometimes reddish, sometimes white.

USES

This is a remedy which may be called for in the many conditions surrounding difficult dentition, particularly in the young dog, especially when there are gastro-intestinal upsets accompanying this. Some forms of white scour in calves may respond especially if associated with nervous symptoms. It should always be considered for suckling animals which reject the mother's milk. It has been found of value in swelling of the mammary glands and could be of use in false pregnancy of the bitch.

Agaricus Muscarius

Toadstool. *N.O.* Fungi. The Ø is prepared from the fresh fungus. Muscarin is the best known toxic compound of several which are found in this fungus. Symptoms of poisoning are generally delayed from anything up to twelve hours after ingestion. The main sphere of action is on the central nervous system producing a state of vertigo and delirium followed by sleepiness. There are four recognised stages of cerebral excitement as follows: 1. Slight stimulation: 2. Intoxication with mental excitement, accompanied by twitching: 3. Delirium with possible crying or screaming: 4. Depression with soporific tendencies.

Head. Vertigo with head in constant motion. Tendency to fall backwards.

Eyes. Twitching of the lids, the margins of which may be inflamed and agglutinated. The inner canthi become red and corneal ulcers may develop. The eyes may assume a narrow appearance.

Skin. Miliary eruptions with swelling. Angio-neurotic oedema.

Alimentary System.   Twitching of mouth with white trembling tongue. Swelling of gums with aphthous ulcers under tongue. Great thirst with difficult swallowing. Diarrhoea accompanies abdominal flatulence.

Respiratory System.   Cough associated with difficult breathing.

Circulatory System.   Pulse weak and intermittent, irregularities being worse in the evening.

Extremities.   There is particular sensitivity over the sacral region. Twitching of various groups of muscles is a fairly constant feature, e.g. of the cervical region, face, ears and eyes. Overall stiffness is common with a tendency to limb paralysis.

Renal System.   Polyuria accompanied by a mucous urethral discharge.

USES

The sphere of action determines its use in certain conditions affecting the central nervous system, e.g. cerebro-cortical necrosis of sheep and cattle and in meningitis which may accompany attacks of hypomagnesaemia in cows. In small animal practice it may be needed in the treatment of post-distemper chorea as well as in eczema showing nervous involvement. Tympanitic conditions with flatus may respond favourably while it also has a place as a rheumatic remedy and for muscular cramp.

Agnus Castus

N.O. Verbenaceae. The Ø is prepared from the ripe berries.

The main action of this plant is in the genital sphere where it causes a diminution in the function of various parts.

Eyes.   Orbital eczema. Pupils dilated. Photophobia.

Alimentary System.   Mouth and gum ulcers. Lack of thirst. Tenderness over abdomen. Splenitis. Ascites.

Renal System.   Output of urine increased.

Male Genital System.   Tendency to impotence.

Female Genital System.   Sterility with yellow-white discharges. Agalactia. Metritis. Retained placenta.

USES

Mainly used in the treatment of particular conditions affecting the genital sphere in both sexes. May give good results in retention of afterbirth if other remedies fail to act.

Ailanthus Glandulosa

Chinese Sumach.   *N.O.* Simarubaceaea. The Ø is prepared from the flowers when they begin to open. The active principle causes conditions met with in low grade septic fevers, especially those showing disruptive skin lesions. There is a tendency to haemorrhages from mucous membranes which become ulcerated. General torpor or prostration is not uncommon.

Eyes. These have a congestive look. Aversion to light with dilated pupils.

Alimentary System. The tongue is dry and cracked. Inflammation of the throat takes the form of an oedematous swelling which is visible from the outside. The teeth are covered with sordes while diarrhoea or dysentery is a usual feature.

Respiratory System. Thin blood-stained nasal discharge with quick irregular breathing. Cough if present is dry and unproductive.

Skin. A periodic miliary rash livid in appearance is occasionally seen. Blisters appear filled with blood-stained serum. The liquid eruptions disappear on pressure.

USES

Certain forms of septic fever may benefit from this remedy, e.g. subacute puerperal metritis following abortion. Mucosal disease of cattle may respond, especially mild forms with oedema of throat and dryness of muzzle which could show bronze-coloured discolouration. Swelling of parotid glands accompanies throat ulceration which may be associated with tenderness over the liver and a watery diarrhoea. It could be useful in thyroid conditions where the gland is swollen and tender. Facial eczema may be helped especially when the eruptions are dark and there is a bleeding from nose and gums.

Aletris Farinosa

Star Grass. *N.O.* Haemodoracae. The Ø is prepared from the root.

This plant exerts its action mainly on the uterus producing a variety of symptoms. There is also a marked action on the stomach and intestines.

Alimentary System. Loss of appetite. Scanty stool with tendency to diarrhoea.

Renal System. Incontinence. Reduced output of urine. Sediment with phosphates.

Female Sexual System. Metrorrhagia, blood dark. Tendency to prolapse. Sterility. Tendency to miscarriage.

USES

A useful remedy in many conditions affecting the uterus, particularly bleeding and discharges of various kinds. It should be remembered as one of the remedies which could influence the infertile state.

Alfalfa

Lucerne. *N.O.* Graminaceae. This plant favourably influences nutrition producing an increase in appetite and digestion. It corrects tissue waste while increasing the quantity and quality of milk in nursing mothers.

Alimentary System. There is increased thirst and appetite while the abdomen becomes flatulent with stools frequent and loose.

Renal System. There is increased urination with frequent urging, the urine showing an increased elimination of phosphates and urea.

USES

Disorders characterised by malnutrition come within its sphere of action. Its action on the urinary system suggests its use in diabetes insipidus and phosphaturia. It might be of use in rheumatic or gouty states of old dogs. One of its main uses in veterinary practice is to increase both the quantity and quality of milk when given in low potency, e.g. lx or Ø. Higher potencies could be used to dry the secretion in conditions such as false pregnancy.

Allium Cepa

Red Onion. *N.O.* Liliaceae. Tincture of the onion or of the whole fresh plant is used. This vegetable produces a picture of coryza with acrid nasal discharge and symptoms of laryngeal discomfort.

Eyes. Redness and inflammation accompany aversion to light and lachrymation. Eyelids are swollen and oedematous.

Respiratory System. Copious, acrid, watery discharge from the nose. Breathing is oppressed and laboured.

Alimentary System. Thirst is prominent. Abdominal tympany with flatus leads to diarrhoea.

Renal System. Tendency to increased urination which produces a reddish sediment.

Extremities. Small joints may be painful producing lesions.

USES

This remedy is indicated in the early stages of most catarrhal conditions producing the typical watery coryza. Mild forms of cat 'flu may be cut short and complications prevented if given frequently as early as possible. Eye conditions generally are helped where the discharge is watery and there is prominence of small blood-vessels. Catarrhal laryngitis may benefit.

Allium Sativum

Garlic. *N.O.* Liliaceae. The Ø is prepared from the fresh bulb. This herb acts directly on the intestinal mucous membrane increasing peristalsis. It also possesses vasodilatory properties.

Eyes. Lachrymation with a tendency for the lids to agglutinate.

Ears. Crusty eruptions appear on the outer ear flap.

Alimentary System. Salivation is a prominent symptom and the appetite is voracious. Papillae of tongue and gums become red. Constipation is usual.

Respiratory System. Mucus collects in the bronchi producing a rattling sound with a loose cough. There may be bleeding from the lungs.

Renal System. The urine is dark brown producing sedimentation.

USES

This remedy should be considered in chronic intestinal affections showing a tendency to colitis and catarrhal inflammations: also in conditions which manifest themselves after a change of food or water. It should be considered in more acute conditions such as mucosal disease and colibacillosis of calves and possibly coccidiosis where it may produce good results if other more indicated remedies fail. The form of mucosal disease showing frothy salivation and a red appearance of the papillae should be particularly helped.

Aloe

Socotrine Aloes. *N.O.* Liliaceae. The Ø is prepared from a solution in spirit of the gum. Where disease and drug symptoms are confused, this remedy is useful in restoring physiological equilibrium. Congestion of the portal circulation is the main result of material doses of this substance.

Alimentary System. The tongue is dry producing a desire for water. The pharyngeal region of the throat is congested with a varicose state of the veins. Abdominal flatulence occurs and pressure over the umbilicus produces pain which is worse over the hepatic region. Straining of rectum is common with jelly-like stools containing mucus.

Renal System. The urine is scanty and high-coloured. Urging to urinate is frequent, particularly at night.

Extremities. Pain and tenderness over the sacral region.

USES

This is a useful remedy to combat allopathic drug dosing. In congestive states of the liver it will help the portal circulation and restore a normal bowel action.

Alumen

Potash Alum. Trituration of the pure crystals is used to prepare the tincture. This substance produces a tendency to induration with the development of ulcers with hard edges. These ulcers frequently become chronic. Bowel symptoms are prominent while there is a tendency to hardening of tissues generally and of the uterus particularly.

Ears. A purulent otorrhoea may arise.

Alimentary System. Various affections of the teeth and gums occur and also a hardening of the tongue. The throat is swollen and red and the tonsils enlarged and indurated. In the dog, cat and pig there is frequent vomiting while in all species obstinate constipation accompanies ineffectual straining.

Female Genital System. The vagina shows aphthous patches. The uterus becomes markedly indurated leading to an acrid discharge. This tendency to induration is also seen in the development of hard lumps in the mammary glands.

Respiratory System. Difficult breathing is associated with bleeding from the lungs.

Skin. Ulcers appear with indurated edges.

Lymphatic System. The lymphatic glands are at first inflamed and later assume the typical hardness associated with this chemical.

Extremities. Great weakness of all muscles is evident particularly in the limbs. This can lead to a staggering gait and incipient paralysis.

USES

The sphere of action of this remedy lies in conditions showing glandular indurations and skin ulcerations showing the specific hard edges. It should be of service in actinobacillosis of cattle and in nodular affections of the mammary gland in bitches. In chronic uterine catarrh of the bitch it could prove useful. Lymphadenoma and Hodgkins Disease may benefit and the remedy is certainly worth a trial in these conditions.

Alumina

Aluminium Oxide. The Ø is prepared from triturations. A condition of dryness of mucous membranes and skin is produced by this substance, while paretic states are common making it a remedy well adapted to old subjects showing debility.

Eyes. Chronic conjunctivitis, aversion to light and lachrymation.

Ears. Dry scurf around the external ear. Otorrhoea is sometimes present.

Alimentary System. Gums become spongy and bleeding is common. Sordes appear on the teeth and throat is dry. A craving for abnormal substances is seen, e.g. charcoal. Rectal activity leads to straining at stool, faeces being hard and knotty.

Renal System. Straining occurs before urination, caused by a paretic condition of the bladder muscle. The urine shows a white sediment.

Extremities. There is a tendency to spinal degeneration with consequent paralysis of the lower limbs. The nails assume a brittle state.

USES

Any condition producing emaciation and vomiting together with weakness of the lower limbs should be helped; also affections showing excessive dryness of mucous membranes and feverish states where the temperature remains elevated. It will be found useful in the early stages of Stuttgart's Disease. Eye conditions producing agglutination of eyelids by night and lachrymation by day should be helped. Skin conditions also benefit where the eruptions are rough and dry and bleed easily assuming a cracked appearance as in various eczematous states.

Ammonium Benzoicum

Benzoate of Ammonia. This salt which is prepared from a solution in distilled water is one of the remedies used for albuminuria with deposits of gouty material in joints.

Eyes. Swollen eyelids with congested look.

Alimentary System. Ranula-like swelling develops under the tongue. Indigestion may arise.

Renal System. Albuminuria with thick deposit on standing. Urine becomes dark and scanty.

Extremities. Tenderness over kidney region, extending to sacrum.

USES

Considering its sphere of action we should think of this remedy in the many kidney ailments affecting dogs, especially those showing deposit of albumen in the urine together with uric acid crystals and a tendency to urinary suppression. It could prove of value in the treatment of ranula.

Ammonium Carbonicum

Carbonate of Ammonia.   Sal Volatile.   This salt is also prepared from
a solution in distilled water. It is used primarily in relation to fat subjects with weak hearts and respiratory affections. There is a tendency to
swollen glands.

Eyes.   Agglutination of eyelids chiefly during night.

Respiratory System.   Coryza with watery nasal discharge.
Epistaxis may occur. Difficult breathing with nightly coughing. Mucus
accumulates in the chest leading to pulmonary oedema.

Alimentary System.   Dryness of mouth and throat with vesicles on tongue. The tonsils become enlarged and sometimes necrotic.
The appetite remains good but is easily satisfied. The abdomen is tympanitic with passage of flatus, accompanied by constipation.

Renal System.   Frequent urination, especially at night. There is
a tendency to diabetes insipidus with whitish urine containing a sandy
deposit.

Skin.   A miliary rash is common with itching and blistery eruption. Eczematous lesions occur in the bends of joints.

Extremities.   The gait is weak because of muscular cramps
making walking difficult.

USES

This remedy is particularly well adapted to thoracic conditions.
Emphysema should benefit while pulmonary oedema and allergic conditions such as fog fever in cattle are just two of many ailments involving
the chest which should respond to its use. Post-influenzal cough accompanying a weak constitution also calls for its use: also chronic bronchitis.
In the alimentary sphere it has been used successfully in flatulent colic
in the horse. In general it is a good constitutional remedy for animals
showing lack of strength with flabby muscles. The urinary symptoms
indicate that it could be of use in threatened diabetic and uraemic
states.

Ammonium Causticum

Hydrate of Ammonia.   Prepared from solution in distilled water. This
salt produces an ulcerative condition of mucous membranes accompanied by oedema. It is also a powerful cardiac stimulant.

Respiratory System.   An ulcerative condition of the nasal
mucosa occurs leading to an excoriating discharge. Respiration is difficult on account of the accumulation of mucus in the chest leading to
coughing.

Alimentary System.   Spasm of the glottis produces a suffocative effect while the abdomen shows flatulence with signs of colic or
unease characterised by kicking at the belly and rolling.
Extremities.   Excessive muscular weakness develops.
Skin.   Becomes hot and dry.

USES

This is another remedy which has been used successfully in the treatment of flatulent colic in the horse. Mucosal disease of calves may
benefit because of the ulcerative state produced on mucous membranes.
Fog fever could also benefit. In pulmonary congestion it is indicated
when there is excess of mucus with a moist cough and muscular weakness, e.g. in some forms of influenza.

Ammonium Muriaticum

Ammonium Chloride.   Sal Ammoniac.   Prepared from dilute solutions. A distinctive quality of this salt is that all mucous secretions are
retained while being increased in quantity. This retention leads to
various catarrhal states such as coughing due to increased activity of the
mucous lining of the bronchi. Many symptoms are accompanied by profuse glairy secretions.
Eyes.   There is a tendency to the development of cataract.
Respiratory System.   Acrid coryza develops with salivation.
Cough is frequent especially after eating, the chest developing a
rattling sound due to the production of mucus.
Alimentary System.   The throat becomes swollen leading to
difficulty in swallowing. The liver becomes congested and signs of
hepatitis may appear, e.g. jaundice and darkening of urine.
Skin.   Pruritus accompanies the development of blisters in various areas.

USES

This is a useful remedy for dogs which have accumulated too much fat
and are lethargic and disinclined for exercise as a result. Certain respiratory conditions showing catarrhal involvement may be helped and in
this connection we should expect to see large amounts of mucus produced in the bronchi and trachea. It may therefore be of use in cat 'flu
and also in fog fever of cattle and in these conditions the catarrhal
secretions are seldom free-flowing when this remedy is indicated.
Digestive upsets showing a sluggish liver function should respond well
when accompanied by respiratory involvement and possibly skin eruptions.

Anacardium Orientale

Marking Nut. *N.O.* Anarcardiaceae. The Ø is prepared from the layer of nut between shell and kernel. Trituration of the dried substance provides the Ø.

In veterinary practice this remedy is not often called for but it may have a place in the treatment of patients showing a diminution in one or other of the special senses, e.g. smell or sight. It also has a strong affinity for the digestive system.

Alimentary System. Vesicles appear in the mouth accompanied by slight bleeding and profuse salivation. Digestion is weak and the abdomen becomes tympanitic with inactive bowels. Spasmodic contraction of the anal sphincter occurs.

Respiratory System. Coughing is produced which is worse after the animal feeds. This symptom is more often seen in cattle than other species.

Cardiac System. Pericarditis sets in accompanied by palpitation.

Extremities. The weakness which arises in the legs may develop gradually to mild paralysis.

Skin. Eczema occurs taking the form of itching vesicular eruptions.

USES

Complaints which appear to be eased by eating may benefit from this remedy, an exception being coughing which often worsens after food. Gradual deterioration of sight accompanying digestive symptoms may benefit.

Anagallis Arvensis

Scarlet Pimpernel. *N.O.* Primulaceae. The Ø is prepared from the whole fresh plant. This plant exerts its main action on the skin producing pruritus. It also favours the expulsion of splinters and can hasten the destruction of warty growths.

Skin. Severe itching is produced which is accompanied by an eruption of dry scales which have been described as 'bran-like'. These are chiefly over the lower limbs and feet. Groups of vesicles may also arise, leading eventually to the formation of ulcers.

Extremities. Discomfort over the shoulder region suggests pain, possibly of rheumatic or gouty origin. Joint swellings may appear.

USES

In veterinary practice this remedy should be considered in the treat-

ment of the particular type of eczema associated with the characteristic
bran-like flakes accompanied by severe itching. It may also prove useful
in the treatment of sessile warts especially in the older animal.

Angustura Vera

N.O. Rutaceae.   The Ø is prepared from trituration of the bark and
subsequent solution in alcohol.
This plant exerts a powerful influence on the musculo-skeletal
system producing bruised and stiff extremities.
Eyes.   Redness with agglutination of eyelids. Eyes appear fixed
and prominent.
Alimentary System.   Dryness of mouth, with later accumulation of thick mucus. Tongue becomes white. Great thirst. Colicky pains
with cramping of abdominal muscles. Borborygmi preceding diarrhoea
contains slimy mucus.
Renal System.   Scanty urination. Urine becomes orange-
coloured.
Extremities.   Stiffness of muscles and joints. Aversion to walking which produces pain. Caries of long bones. Cracking in joints.

USES
A useful remedy for controlling some forms of arthritis in older dogs.
Has been used successfully in bone spavin and obscure cases of joint
cracking. The action of the alimentary canal suggests that it could be of
use in white scour of calves.

Antimonium Crudum

Black Antimony Sulphide.   The Ø is prepared from triturations. This
substance produces skin conditions which are aggravated by heat.
Eyes.   There is a dull look in the eye. Swelling of the eyelids produces a sunken look. The lids themselves become agglutinated and corneal pustules may occur.
Ears.   Moist eruptions occur on and behind ears accompanied by
redness and swelling. Various types of discharge occur.
Respiratory System.   Paroxysms of coughing take place with
expectoration of mucus. Eczematous lesions appear around the nostrils.
Alimentary System.   The tongue is thickly coated with whitish
exudate which appears as salivation of slimy mucus when excessive.
Appetite is poor. The margins of the gums show bleeding where they
join the teeth. In the dog, cat and pig vomiting occurs. Flatulence

occurs in all species with possibly diarrhoea. In contrast to the lack of appetite, thirst may be excessive.

Urinary System.   There is frequency of urination, the urine being turbid and albuminous and of a deep golden-brown colour.

Extremities.   Dogs may show the development of warty excrescenses on the skin of the pads. There is generalised twitching of muscles.

Skin.   Complaints of gastric origin are frequently associated with eczema which takes the form of urticaria with miliary eruptions. The skin remains dry with a tendency to wart formation while vesicles occur which soon develop into ulcers containing a honey-like secretion.

USES

This is a useful remedy in the treatment of eczematous and nephritic conditions of the dog and cat, possibly associated with stomach disorders. The effect on the pads of dogs suggests its use in distemper associated with scaling and hardening. Blepharitis and conjunctivitis may benefit. It has been used successfully in the treatment of the early stages of cow pox and will prevent development of the lesions. It could be of benefit in the treatment of vesicular stomatitis in all species.

Antimonium Tartaricum

Tartar Emetic.   The Ø is prepared from triturations. Respiratory symptoms predominate with this substance, affections being accompanied by the production of excess mucus, although expectoration is difficult.

Alimentary System.   The tongue is coated, with red edges. Swallowing is difficult and is accompanied by retching. Vomiting may take place in the dog, cat and pig. Spasmodic bouts of colicky pain occur in all species, characterised by abdominal kicking and rumbling. This symptom is worse before stool which is accompanied by straining. The stools are watery and contain mucus.

Respiratory System.   There is great production of mucus which produces a rattling sound in the chest. Expectoration is slight but there may be a frothy saliva. The abundance of mucus may lead to pulmonary oedema followed by emphysema with short rapid breathing.

Urinary System.   The urine is scanty, strong-smelling and dark. Haematuria and cystitis may be present.

Extremities.   Twitching of muscles accompanies tenderness over the lumbo-sacral region.

Skin.   Pustular eruptions occur with a tendency to wart formation, but this is less common than with antimony crudum.

Circulatory System.   Pulse is rapid and weak. Auscultation reveals a fluttering action.

USES

The main action being exerted in the respiratory sphere, we should expect this remedy to be of use in conditions such as broncho-pneumonia and pulmonary oedema and it has won many laurels in this respect. Such symptoms accompany fog fever in cattle and the remedy has given good results in the treatment of this condition. Ailments requiring this remedy may show drowsiness and thirstlessness. In pneumonic conditions the edges of the eyes may be agglutinated by mucus.

Antipyrene

Phenazone. The Ø is prepared from solutions or triturations. This substance induces leucocytosis. It acts especially on the vasomotor centre causing dilation of skin capillaries leading to hyperaemia and swelling.

Head. Oedema and puffiness occur producing a heavy swollen appearance.

Alimentary System. The swelling already mentioned extends to the lips. The tongue shows ulceration, lesions leading to the formation of throat abscesses.

Urinary System. Output of urine is reduced and in extreme cases may be completely suppressed.

Respiratory System. Oppression of breathing occurs due to a degree of pulmonary oedema.

Skin. The capillary dilation leads to a state of erythema with possibly angio-neurotic oedema. Eczema and urticaria are common accompaniments.

USES

Because of its leucocytic action this remedy may benefit mild cases of Hodgkins's Disease. Angio-neurotic oedema will also come within its sphere of action. The early symptoms of uraemia may be relieved by the use of a high potency to promote diuresis.

Apis Mellifica

Honey Bee Venom. The Ø is prepared from the whole bee, subsequent dilutions being dissolved in alcohol.

The poison of the bee acts on cellular tissue causing oedema of skin and subcutaneous tissue and results in puffiness and swelling. The production of oedema anywhere in the system may lead to a variety of acute and chronic conditions.

Eyes.   Eyelids become swollen and oedematous producing a heavy paralysed look. Conjunctivitis sets in and there is strong aversion to light.

Head.   Ears become swollen and there is an enlarged appearance of all tissue.

Alimentary System.   The oedema which arises in the throat creates difficulty in swallowing. The tongue also shows swelling. Abdominal dropsy occurs and may be due to many factors. Stools are usually brown and watery.

Urinary System.   Acute nephritis with scanty burning urine is commonly seen. This is accompanied by cast formation. Suppression of urine may occur. Haematuria with albuminuria is seen in hyperacute cases.

Respiratory System.   Oedema in the lungs leads to difficulty in breathing. This extends to the laryngeal area causing retching with salivation.

Circulatory System.   The heart action is feeble with intermittent pulse and the cardiac region is painful on touch. On auscultation there is a rasping sound which accompanies the contraction of heart muscle.

Extremities.   In the horse and cow there may be oedema of lower limbs while in dogs abdominal dropsy is seen. In all species the carpal and tarsal joints become swollen and tender.

Skin.   The skin may assume an erysipeloid appearance due to oedematous swelling.

USES

Considering the well-documented evidence of its sphere of action affecting all tissues and mucous membranes we should remember this remedy in the treatment of conditions showing oedema. It is valuable in the early stages of actue nephritis. Synovial swellings of joints will benefit. Fog fever with its abundance of respiratory mucus has been treated successfully with this remedy. Cystic ovaries may also respond. All ailments are aggravated by heat and unaccompanied by thirst. Joint conditions such as bog spavin, thoroughpin and acute navicular disease may show encouraging results. In nephritis with suppression it has been known to promote copious urination.

Apocynum Cannabinum

Indian Hemp.   *N.O.* Apocynaceae.   The Ø is prepared from the whole fresh plant including the root. This plant acts on cellular tissue producing a dropsical condition increasing the secretion of mucous and serous membranes. One of its main effects is to reduce the pulse rate.

Eyes. Lachrymation results from irritation and inflammation of eye structures.

Alimentary System. An increase of mucus in the mouth produces salivation in the dog, cat and pig. There may be vomiting, food and water being immediately rejected. Ascites occurs with bloating.

Urinary System. Difficult urination occurs but the amount of urine is increased. This is due to bladder distension, the contents gradually being added to due to poor expulsive powers of the bladder musculature. The urine contains a thick mucus of a yellow colour.

Respiratory System. Nasal catarrh is seen, the secretion being thick and yellow. Cough is usually present.

Cardiac System. The heart action is feeble and irregular with low arterial tension. This leads to generalised dropsy.

Extremities. In the horse and cow oedema of the lower limbs and brisket occurs.

USES

This is a useful remedy in cardiac cases showing the characteristic oedema in various parts. Also in renal and bladder insufficiency accompanying digestive upsets. In the dog diabetes insipidus has been treated successfully. It will also promote urination both by stimulating the heart's action and by toning up the musculature of the bladder.

Apomorphinum

Apomorphine Hydrochloride. The Ø is prepared from a solution in distilled water.

This substance has a profound action on the vomiting centre giving rise to emesis without accompanying nausea. Drowsy and faint states accompany this.

USES

It is used solely in veterinary practice for repeated vomiting in the dog, cat or pig and may produce excellent results where other remedies fail.

Argentum Metallicum

Metallic Silver. The Ø is prepared from trituration. The main action of this element is centred on articulations and component parts, bones, ligaments and cartilages. Carious affections result from small blood-vessels becoming atrophied.

Eyes. Eyelids become thickened and red. Photophobia and a purulent opthalmia may arise, usually worse in the young animal.

Ears.   Itching and scratching are common features.

Respiratory System.   Fluent nasal catarrh occurs while the laryngeal area is severly inflamed. Cough, if present, is dry and unproductive.

Alimentary System.   The appearance of the tongue suggests dryness but actually salivation is common. This produces a jelly-like mucus which makes swallowing difficult. Appetite remains good. There is rumbling of flatus with dry stools.

Urinary System.   Urine is increased, the urine being turbid and sweet-smelling.

Extremities.   Rheumatic-like affections of joints are common especially affecting the carpus and elbow. Sub-maxillary swellings lead to stiffness of the cervical region while there is pain and tenderness over the pelvis.

USES

This is a useful remedy in joint stiffness of the older dog. Some digestive conditions may benefit, especially those in prematurely aged animals.

Argentum Nitricum

Silver Nitrate.   The Ø is prepared from trituration. This salt produces incoordination of movement and loss of balance. Symptoms of central nervous system disturbance predominate causing trembling in various parts. It has an irritant effect on mucous membranes producing a free-flowing muco-purulent discharge. Red blood-cells are affected, anaemia being caused by their destruction.

Eyes.   The inner canthus becomes red and swollen. Various complications arise leading to purulent ophthalmia and corneal opacity with ulceration. There is strong aversion to light.

Respiratory System.   Difficult oppressive coughing takes place.

Alimentary System.   The mouth is sensitive and tender. Canker sores occur leading to bleeding from the gums. Gastro-enteritis is usual accompanied by abdominal bloating and diarrhoea after eating and drinking. Involvement of the stomach leads to vomiting in the dog, cat and pig.

Urinary System.   There is a tendency to suppression, the urine being dark and scanty. The irritant effect on mucous membranes may produce a urethritis when the urine contains purulent material.

Extremities.   Trembling occurs in all limbs and in severe cases there may be slight paralysis.

Male Genital System.   The sexual organs become withered and shrivelled-looking.

Skin. In light skinned animals a bronze or dark discolouration occurs.

USES

Many chronic complaints of old animals come within its sphere of action, e.g. gastric and intestinal affections which heal and then relapse. Eye conditions are especially benefited, e.g. ophthalmia, cataract and corneal opacities and ulceration. Anaemia will also improve. The action on the central nervous system enables one to prescribe this remedy for those animals exhibiting fears and nervousness especially towards other animals.

Arnica Montana

Leopard's Bane. *N.O.* Compositae. The Ø is prepared from the whole fresh plant. The action of this plant upon the body is practically synonymous with a state resulting from injuries or blows. It is known as the 'Fall Herb' and is found growing in mountainous regions. It has a marked affinity with blood-vessels leading to dilation, stasis and increased permeability. Thus various types of haemorrhage can occur.

Eyes. Subconjunctival and retinal haemorrhages occur giving a reddish, bruised appearance.

Respiratory System. Nasal bleeding of dark fluid blood occurs. Severe coughing accompanies pneumonia which affects principally the right lung.

Alimentary System. Hunger is constant but food is rejected. Gastric bleeding may occur. The haemorrhagic tendency extends to the large intestine leading to dysenteric stools accompanied by colicky pains and much straining.

Urinary System. Retention of urine is usual while there is difficulty in expulsion due to weakness of the bladder wall.

Cardiac System. The heart becomes enlarged while a generalised cardiac dropsy appears.

Skin. Miliary eruptions give a bruised appearance. Purpura and ecchymoses are common features as also are small boils with a tendency to become septic and putrid.

USES

The well proven symptoms of poisoning by this plant determine its use in all conditions where bruising and injury occur and where the skin remains unbroken. It reduces shock and should be a routine prescription before and after surgical interference, including tooth extractions. Given after parturition it will hasten recovery of bruised tissues while its use during pregnancy will lessen the danger of difficult labour. It is of use in retinal and other eye haemorrhages, while as a heart remedy it restores tone to a weakened muscle. Arnica may also be used externally as a liniment in the treatment of sprained or bruised tendons and muscles.

Arsenicum Album

Arsenic Trioxide.   The Ø is prepared from triturations. This deeply-acting element acts on every tissue of the body and its characteristic and definite symptoms make its use certain in many ailments. Restlessness is a key symptom, the patient frequently changing position. Symptoms of fear are also prominent and are exacerbated towards midnight. Discharges are acrid and burning and symptoms are relieved by heat.

Eyes.   Lachrymation with red ulcerated lids. Corneal ulceration.

Respiratory System.   Severe acrid coryza occurs producing scabs around the nostrils. Coughing and wheezing respiration are associated with bleeding from the lungs.

Cardiac System.   Auscultation reveals a rapid palpitating pulse.

Alimentary System.   The mouth is dry with ulceration of gums. The throat is swollen and oedematous. Vomiting occurs in the dog, cat and pig and may be blood-stained. Thirst is prominent but the amounts taken at any one time are small. Abdominal swelling occurs due in part to swelling of liver and spleen which leads to ascites. Inflammation of the lower bowel produces a picture of straining and tenesmus with dysenteric stools of a cadaverous odour.

Urinary System.   Bright's Disease occurs producing albuminuria with casts. The bladder may become paralysed leading to difficulty in expelling urine.

Skin.   This is usually dry and scaly with persistent itching and loss of hair. There may be eruptions while oedema of subcutaneous tissues is seen in severe cases.

Male Genital System.   Orchitis occurs along with swelling of scrotal skin.

Extremities.   Peripheral neuritis arises leading to loss of nutrition of affected parts. This results in withering and eventual gangrene, preceded by extreme pruritus. This causes the animal to bite vigorously at the affected parts.

USES

The all-embracing sphere of action of this remedy makes its use in practice essential in many well-defined conditions, e.g. canine distemper and feline enteritis. It is also of use in dry eczema where the skin condition is accompanied by the production of flakes like dandruff. A characteristic symptom which is seen in most conditions is thirst for small quantities of water together with an aggravation of symptoms towards midnight. In addition animals are restless frequently changing their positions. Most ailments are improved by warmth. In the horse it has given good results in sweet itch. In cattle practice it is a most useful remedy in the control of some forms of calf scour where the stool has a cadaverous odour and is accompanied by severe straining. Respiratory conditions which show the typical arsenicum symptoms will also benefit. It has a specific action in swine dysentery and in gastro-enteric conditions generally will quickly allay vomiting and diarrhoea provided the characteristic symptoms overall predominate.

Arsenicum Iodatum

Arsenic Iodide.   The Ø is prepared from triturations. When discharges are persistently irritating and corrosive, this remedy may prove of more value than Arsenicum Album. Muçus membranes become red, swollen and oedematous, especially in the respiratory sphere.

Alimentary System.   Pharyngitis occurs with swollen tonsils. There is persistent vomiting and intense thirst.

Eyes.   Ophthalmia is seen with corrosive discharge. Severe corneal ulceration accompanies most conditions.

Ears.   Chronic otitis externa with discharge of acrid material which excoriates the ear flap.

Respiratory System.   Thin, watery burning discharges take place. Bronchitis and chronic pneumonia with persistent cough are frequently seen.

Skin.   This is usually dry and scaly with itching and exfoliation.

USES

It is of use in much the same conditions which call for Arsenicum Album but may be of more use in bronchial and pneumonic illness which does not properly respond to other more indicated remedies. It is a good convalescent remedy after influenza and pneumonia. Ear canker in the dog frequently responds well.

Baptisia Tinctoria

Wild Indigo. *N.O.* Leguminosae. The Ø is prepared from the fresh root and its bark.

The symptoms produced by this plant relate mainly to septicaemic conditions involving prostration and weakness. Low grade fevers and great muscular lethargy are present in the symptomatology. All secretions and discharges are very offensive.

Alimentary System. Profuse salivation is present with offensive breath and mouth ulceration, which accompanies a yellow-brown discolouration of tongue and gums. Tonsils and throat are dark red, the inflammation making swallowing difficult. In the dog, cat and pig vomiting occurs, while gastro-enteritis is common in all species. Stools are dysenteric.

Extremities. Muscular weakness is accompanied by stiffness and signs of discomfort and possibly also of pain.

Skin. Ulceration occurs with putrid discharges.

USES

The action of this remedy makes its homoeopathic use worthy of consideration in many conditions giving rise to a low-grade form of septicaemia, e.g. after abortion when metritis may arise. It may also be indicated in salmonellosis and Stuttgart's Disease. Influenza in the horse accompanied by lethargy and weakness may respond well especially if there is abdominal involvement also. Certain manifestations of canine distemper, e.g. those exhibiting putrid discharges will also benefit.

Baryta Carbonica

Barium Carbonate with Acetate. The Ø is prepared from trituration and dilution in distilled water. The action of this substance produces symptoms and conditions which are of importance mainly in the very young and the very old.

Respiratory System. There is nasal discharge which tends to

dry quickly giving the nostrils a caked appearance. Cough when present
is also dry and unproductive and is worse on inspiration.

Alimentary System. There is a tendency to bleeding from
gums with inflamed vesicles in the mouth. Sub-maxillary glands become
swollen and may show suppuration. Abdominal tympany may occur.

Cardiac System. The heart's action is at first accelerated
giving a tense pulse which later becomes involved.

USES

This remedy should be remembered when dealing with conditions in
animals at the extremes of life. It could prove of value e.g. in the treatment of bronchial conditions in suckling animals and also in tensive
states in the older subject.

Balsamum Peruvianum

Balsam of Peru.   *N.O.* Leguminosae.   The Ø is prepared from the
balsam that flows from the stems.

This substance produces bronchial catarrhal symptoms with purulent expectoration.

Respiratory System.   The main symptom is bronchitis leading
to catarrhal involvement of the upper respiratory tract. There is a loose
cough and loud râles can be heard on auscultation.

Urinary System.   The urine is scanty and contains a mucous
sediment dependent on a catarrhal cystitis.

Alimentary System.   In the dog, cat and pig vomiting occurs of
mucoid catarrhal material.

USES

This remedy is useful as a stimulant to raw surfaces promoting granulation of wounds and ulcers and helping to keep mucous surfaces dry. It is
of value in catarrhal states of the respiratory tract. Chronic forms of
pyelitis and cystitis may benefit.

Belladonna

Deadly Nightshade.   *N.O.* Solanaceae.   The entire plant at flowering
is used in the preparation of the Ø.

Belladonna produces a profound action on every part of the nervous system causing a state of excitement and active congestion. The
effect on the skin, glands and vascular system is specific.

Central Nervous System.   Delirium occurs with biting and severe head shaking. There is unsteadiness of gait with a tendency to fall backwards or sideways, and the head may roll from side to side. Twitching of neck and throat muscles is seen.

Eyes.   The pupils are markedly dilated and in severe cases there may be protrusion of the eye. Conjunctivae become inflamed leading to lachrymation with aversion to light. The animal assumes a fixed staring look.

Ears.   Inflammation of all structures causes the patient to shake the head and in severe cases to knock it against fixed objects. This may take the form of boring the head into a corner.

Respiratory System.   Nose-bleed occurs with bright red blood. Breathing is oppressed and rapid with blood-stained expectoration.

Alimentary System.   Mouth and throat are red with swollen papillae. Swelling of throat makes swallowing difficult. Thirst is prominent with colicky pains and possibly abdominal tympany.

Glandular System.   All glands show swelling and tenderness. This includes the mammary glands.

Urinary System.   Retention of urine with straining to pass. Urine is dark and turbid due to the presence of blood-stained casts.

Extremities.   Joints become swollen, hard and shiny. Great pain is present but little or no increase in joint fluid.

Skin.   Usually dry. Generalised redness and heat. The animal resents touch.

USES

Considering its all-embracing action, this remedy is useful in many conditions in various species. One of the main guiding symptoms is a full, bounding pulse in any feverish condition which may or may not accompany excitability. In cattle the acute form of mastitis occurring after parturition will respond when the udder is hot, tense and swollen. Laminitis in the acute form calls for its use along with Aconitum. In conditions involving the central nervous system such as hypomagnesaemia and some forms of milk fever its early use will help prevent brain damage. Hysteria and fits of various kinds in dogs usually show a good response. This includes the specific form of eclampsia in the bitch, and also those associated with canine distemper. It could also be of use in heat stroke.

Bellis Perennis

The Daisy.   *N.O.* Compositae.   The Ø is prepared from the whole fresh plant. The main action of the daisy is on the muscular fibres of blood-vessels producing a state of venous congestion. Muscles become heavy giving rise to a halting type of gait suggestive of pain or discomfort.

Skin. The congestion causes swelling and exudation and small petechial haemorrhages may develop. Pustular eruptions like small boils are not uncommon.

Female Genital System. Engorgement of uterus may take place due to a generalised pelvic congestion. This may show as uterine bleeding. Mammary glands are swollen and sensitive.

Extremities. The animal is unwilling to move and when made to do so evinces pain. Muscular stiffness is prominent.

USES

Bellis is a useful remedy for aiding bruised tissues, including post-operative states. Sprains and bruises come within its sphere of action (c.f. Arnica). Given post-partum it will hasten resolution of bruised tissue and reduce bleeding. Erysipeloid conditions of the skin may require it.

Benzenum

Benzene. The Ø is prepared from solution in alcohol.

This chemical agent has a marked action on the circulatory system producing a decrease in red and an increase in white cell formation.

Central Nervous System. Epileptiform fits occur leading to coma.

Eyes. Aversion to light with twitching of eyelids and dilation of pupils.

Respiratory System. Fluent nasal catarrh.

Male Genital System. Swelling of testicles may occur with an accompanying scrotal eczema.

Skin. Papular eruptions arise which cause the animal to bite and scratch.

USES

This remedy could possibly be of value in the early stages of Hodgkin's Disease in the dog and cat. It may also be indicated in conditions of the central nervous system producing fits. Orchitis of unknown origin may also respond.

Benzoicum Acidum

Benzoic Acid. The Ø is prepared from solution in distilled water.

The most outstanding action of this acid upon the system relates to the urinary tract, producing changes in the colour and odour of the urine. There is also a marked metabolic action.

Central Nervous System.   Incoordination of movement occurs caused by involvement of the brain. This may cause the animal to fall sideways. In the cat there may be excitability.

Alimentary System.   Ulceration of tongue with bleeding from the gums. A frothy diarrhoea occurs which is light-coloured and has a marked uriniferous odour.

Respiratory System.   Coughing takes place increasing in frequency at night.

Urinary System.   Urine becomes dark with an aromatic odour. The reaction is strongly acid and there are uric acid deposits. Output of urine is reduced while the changes in the kidney extend to the bladder leading to cystitis.

Extremities.   Uric acid deposits occur also in the joints which make a cracking sound on movement. The Achilles tendon is especially sensitive to touch.

Skin.   Itching, red eruptions occur.

USES

The remedy is of value in conditions showing a uric acid diathesis, commonly seen in old dogs, a main guiding symptom being the dark colour and aromatic odour of the urine. Threatened uraemia may be averted, other symptoms being equal. Hysterical and excitable conditions in the cat may benefit.

Berberis Vulgaris

Barberry.   *N.O.* Berberidaceae.   The bark of the root provides the basis of the Ø preparation.

This shrub, of wide distribution, has an affinity with most tissues. Symptoms which arise are liable to alternate quickly, e.g. feverish conditions with thirst can quickly give way to prostration without any desire for water. It acts forcibly on the venous system producing engorgements most frequently seen in the pelvic region.

Eyes.   Various congestive conditions arise leading to ophthalmia.

Respiratory System.   The main effect is on the nasal passages producing a dried mucous membrane.

Alimentary System.   Redness and swelling of the throat occur especially over the tonsillar area. Bile is increased because of a stimulant effect on the liver. In extreme cases this may lead to interference with liver function producing symptoms of jaundice and hepatitis. There may also be an accompanying enteritis giving rise to diarrhoea or dysentery. Stools are mostly clay-coloured.

Urinary System.   Polyuria may alternate with diminished output of urine, which contains mucus and has a reddish tinge.

Extremities. Tenderness occurs over the sacral and pelvic regions with stiffness of associated muscles. Weakness and heaviness of limbs takes place sometimes leading to a disinclination to rise.

Skin. Involvement of skin takes the form of a pustular eczema with pigmentation and a tendency to wart formation.

USES

This is an important remedy in small animal and equine practice. The chief ailments which relate to it are those which show liver and kidney dysfunction. These may lead to catarrhal involvement of bile-ducts, kidney, pelvis and bladder. Jaundice with clay-coloured faeces is a common feature of conditions requiring its use while haematuria and cystitis may respond well if the origin of the trouble is kidney sluggishness. In all conditions there is sacral weakness and tenderness over the loins. It has been used successfully in the treatment of azoturia in the horse and in conditions which give rise to sand and gravel in the urine.

Beryllium

The Metal. The Ø is prepared from trituration and subsequent solution in distilled water.

This metal acts mainly on the respiratory system and to a lesser extent on the skin.

Respiratory System. The changes here are confined mainly to the thoracic cavity producing a variety of conditions ranging from cough to bronchitis, pneumonia and emphysema. All conditions are made worse by exertion.

Alimentary System. Ulcers develop on the tip of the tongue and lips. The throat is red, shiny and glazed looking. In the dog, cat and pig there may be vomiting.

Skin. Papules develop early and grow into ulcers or granulomata, accompanied by intense itching.

USES

This remedy is valuable in the treatment of certain conditions of the chest where the leading indication is difficult breathing even on slight exertion, together with coughing. Auscultation may reveal little change. Both acute and chronic emphysema may benefit. It could also be of use in virus pneumonia, secondary fog fever and chronic bronchitis. In most conditions where it is called for symptoms are few when the animal is at rest, but distress is obvious on movement.

Bismuthum

Bismuth Sub-Nitrate. The Ø is prepared from trituration and subsequent solution in distilled water.

The main action of this chemical centres on the alimentary system, producing catarrhal inflammation of various parts.

Alimentary System. A swollen appearance of the mouth accompanies spongy-looking gums and tongue. Copious saliva is produced. In the dog, cat and pig severe vomiting occurs, water especially being rejected. Gastritis occurs in all species and diarrhoea sets in with rumbling of flatus.

Urinary System. Frequency of urination takes place with also increase in volume of urine.

Extremities. Paralytic weakness of hind-limbs, possibly due to cramping of muscles. The tibial region particularly is tender to the touch.

USES

Gastro-enteric conditions of small animals come within its scope. Polyuria may also benefit other symptoms being equal.

Boracicum Acidum

Boracic Acid. The Ø is prepared from solution of crystals in alcohol.

This acid is capable of arresting fermentation and putrefaction and generally has antiseptic properties.

Eyes. Oedematous swelling of eyes and lids. Conjunctivitis with aversion to light.

Alimentary System. The tongue becomes red, dry and cracked. Saliva is cold to the touch. Inflammation of the pancreas has been noted.

Skin. Redness and swelling occurs in the skin of the upper parts of the body and limbs. Cellulitis occurs around the eyes. Exfoliation of skin takes place as a result of dermatitis.

Urinary System. Frequency of urination accompanies straining to pass.

USES

Eye conditions leading to conjunctivitis will benefit if given early. Pancreatitis in the dog may benefit especially when accompanied by renal symptoms such as polyuria. Orbital cellulitis and eczema of the upper areas should also be remembered in treatment.

Borax

Sodium Biborate.   The Ø is prepared from trituration and subsequent solution in distilled water.

This salt produces gastro-intestinal irritation with mouth symptoms of ulceration and salivation. With most complaints there is an accompanying fear of downward motion.

Central Nervous System.   The animal shows nervousness with an anxious expression and is sensitive to sudden noise.

Eyes.   Generalised inflammation occurs. Entropion frequently arises.

Respiratory System.   Scabs occur around the nostrils giving rise to a mucoid discharge. Difficulty of breathing accompanies a frequent cough.

Alimentary System.   Aphthous ulcers appear in the mouth producing a copious saliva. Distension of appetite may be seen and vomiting occurs in the dog, cat and pig. Catarrhal enteritis leads to a mucoid diarrhoea.

Extremities.   Ulcers appear on the feet, seen in cattle as vesicular involvement of the interdigital cleft. In the dog and cat eczema of the toes leads to loss of nails and claws.

Skin.   Redness and swelling are first seen and suppurative lesions may appear later due to secondary infection.

USES

The specific action of this chemical on the epithelium of the mouth and its ability to cause vesicular eruption on the feet, singles it out as the chief non-biological prophylactic remedy in the control of foot and mouth disease. This has been well documented in various outbreaks and is of great value when used properly. Enteric forms of mucosal disease may also benefit. It is of value in controlling the nervousness exhibited by gun-shy dogs. Mild forms of entropion have yielded successfully to treatment using different potencies. A prominent guiding symptom is fear of downward motion. This will probably be present in the majority of cases where the remedy is indicated.

Bothrops Lanceolatus

Yellow Viper.   The Ø is prepared from solution of the venom in glycerine.

This venom is associated with first, haemorrhages and secondly rapid coagulation of blood. Septic conditions usually supervene after a bite.

Eyes.   Conjunctival and retinal haemorrhages occur. Dim sight.

Alimentary System.   The mouth and throat are dry and swollen making swallowing difficult. Blood-stained vomiting occur in dog, cat and pig while haemorrhagic gastro-enteritis is seen in all species. Abdominal tympany and dysentery are usual.

Skin.   A swollen appearance accompanies a tendency to haemorrhagic infiltration.

Circulatory System.   Haemorrhages may occur from any body orifice and the lymphatic vessels become swollen and tense.

Respiratory System.   Pulmonary oedema and congestion.

USES

This is a valuable remedy in controlling septic states accompanying haemorrhages. Gangrenous conditions of the skin may be prevented by its early use after a bite or in conditions showing similar symptoms. Pulmonary congestions and various types of paralyses come within its orbit. The effects of a bite frequently appear on the opposite limb or part of the body to that bitten. Iliac thrombosis may show improvement (c.f. other snake venoms).

Bovista

Warted Puff Ball.   *N.O.* Fungi.   The Ø is prepared by trituration of the fungus.

This plant has a marked action on the skin producing an eczematous eruption. The circulation is also involved leading to haemorrhages.

Respiratory System.   There is nasal discharge of stringy mucus which produces a scurfy deposit on the nostrils.

Alimentary System.   Bleeding from gums, colic and restlessness are seen, these symptoms being relieved by eating. Constipation is followed by watery diarrhoea with great straining.

Urinary System.   The urine is usually tinged red.

Skin.   Urticarial eczema occurs, at first moist but leading to the formation of crusts. The head is particularly affected with severe itching made worse by warmth. Itching may lead to surface bleeding.

Extremities.   Great weakness affects all joints with tenderness over the sacrum.

Female Genital System.   Bleeding takes place from the uterus. Cystic ovaries can occur, while a greenish-white discharge sets in after oestrus.

USES

This is one of the foremost remedies in the control of eczema in the small animals, particularly when affecting the head. Severe itching is always present. Affections of the female genital tract may also benefit if other characteristic symptoms are present.

Bromium

Bromine.   The Ø is prepared from solution of the element in distilled water.

This element is found in combination with iodine in the ash when seaweed is burnt, and also in sea water. It acts chiefly on the mucous membrane of the respiratory tract, especially the upper trachea causing laryngeal spasm.

Alimentary System.   The throat becomes red and swollen, while inspiration brings on coughing. Pulmonary oedema is present in severe cases.

Glandular and Lymphatic Systems.   Swelling and induration of lymphatic glands occurs, developing slowly. The sub-maxillary and the retropharyngeal glands are chiefly involved. Suppuration does not normally supervene.

Extremities.   Limbs become weak and cold and may show wasting of muscle.

Skin.   Blistering is a fairly constant feature, accompanied by redness and heat.

USES

This is a useful remedy in respiratory conditions of the upper tract which produce a croup-like cough with loose mucus. Symptoms are worse on inspiration. Lymphadenitis of the throat glands should benefit. Eczema which takes the form of a hot blistery rash may need this remedy. Conditions are generally worsened by heat.

Bryonia Alba

White Bryony.   *N.O.* Cucurbitaceae.   The Ø is prepared from the root before flowering takes place.

This important plant produces a glucoside capable of producing severe purgation. The plant itself exerts its main action on epithelial tissues and also on serous and synovial membranes. Some mucous surfaces are affected producing an inflammatory reaction. Exudates become serous and then fibrinous. This in turn leads to dryness of the affected tissue with later effusions into synovial cavities. Movement of parts is interfered with, giving rise to one of its main indications for its use, viz. all symptoms are worse from movement.

Eyes.   There is a tendency to glaucoma.

Respiratory System. Nasal discharges may show bleeding. There is a dry hacking cough with a desire to breathe deeply. The pleural surfaces are particularly involved leading to extensive inflammation.

Alimentary System. The mouth is dry and the animal drinks large quantities. A yellowish deposit covers the tongue and vomiting occurs in the dog, cat and pig. The liver is affected leading to hepatitis and jaundice causing swelling and tenderness over the liver area. In chronic conditions stools become hard and dry.

Urinary System. The urine becomes dark brown and may show turbidity with a pinkish deposit on standing.

Cardiac System. Pericarditis occurs due to extension from the pleura.

Extremities. Joints become swollen and painful, most noticeable in the larger joints like hock and carpus.

USES

This remedy is extremely useful in the treatment of many conditions where a main guiding symptom is worse from movement, e.g. in pneumonia or pleurisy it will be found that the animal prefers to lie on the affected side, bringing pressure to bear and thus restricting movement. Synovitis and joint swellings generally may need this remedy. Mastitis in cattle where the gland remains hard after treatment will probably benefit.

Bufo

Poison of the Toad. The Ø is prepared from solution of the poison in rectified spirit.

The venom of the toad acts on the nervous system and the skin. There is also an action on the lymphatics and the uterus as well as interference with normal muscle movement.

Central Nervous System. Disturbances of normal behaviour take place leading to a disposition to bite. In the dog barking may change to howling and the animal seeks solitude.

Respiratory System. Nose bleeding may occur.

Female Genital System. Hard nodules develop on the mammary glands and the milk of nursing mothers may contain blood. Venous engorgement of pelvic blood-vessels leads to uterine haemorrhage.

Extremities. Cramping of muscles produces a staggering gait.

Skin. Slight injuries lead to pustula eruptions and blisters are commonly seen on the pads of dogs and cats. There is a tendency to suppuration seen in the development of boils, carbuncles and septic lymphangitis.

USES

Conditions of a low septic nature come within its sphere of action, e.g. sub-acute blood-poisoning. Blood in milk post-partum may require it. Mammary nodules in the bitch have been removed by this remedy, other symptoms being equal. Nervous animals and those averse to company may benefit. Metrorrhagia of venous blood may call for this remedy.

Cactus Grandiflorus

Night-blooming Cereus. *N.O.* Cactaceae. The Ø is prepared from young stems and flowers.

The active principle of this plant acts on circular muscle fibres and has a marked affinity for the cardio-vascular system.

Respiratory System. Changes produced are mainly of a haemorrhagic character, e.g. epistaxis and bleeding from lungs.

Alimentary System. Gastro-enteritis, possibly haemorrhagic, is seen. In the dog, cat and pig vomiting occurs while dysentery occurs in all species.

Urinary System. Output of urine is increased, the urine containing varying amounts of blood.

Cardiac System. The changes in the heart are confined to the inner lining leading to endocarditis and valvular insufficiency. Pulse is feeble and irregular.

Extremities. The weakness of the heart's action leads to oedema of various parts. In the dog and cat this occurs as ascites while swelling of the lower limbs and brisket occurs in horses and cattle.

USES

In veterinary practice it has been used in the treatment of valvular disease in the older dog and as a heart stimulant generally.

Calcarea Carbonica

Impure Calcium Carbonate. The Ø is prepared from trituration and subsequent solution in distilled water.

This remedy is prepared from the calcareous substance found in the middle layer of the oyster shell. It produces a lack of tone and muscular weakness muscle spasm affecting both voluntary and involuntary muscle. Calcium is an element which is rapidly excreted and its intake in the crude state does not ensure against certain conditions where it is needed. Calcium is dependent on the presence of sodium, potassium and magnesium in the system before it can be utilised properly and these elements must be in equilibrium.

Eyes.   Dilation of pupils occurs early while progressive deterioration of structures may lead to cataract. Lachrymal glands become easily blocked and the eye assumes an injected inflamed appearance. Ophthalmia may supervene.

Ears.   Discharges of various kinds occur. A cracking sound is sometimes heard when the animal chews.

Alimentary System.   Various conditions may arise in the mouth ranging from tonsillitis to parotid fistula and ranula. Throat glands are enlarged and there is a tendency to umbilical hernia in the young animal. Appetite is frequently depraved.

Skeletal System.   Disorders of bone metabolism occur, e.g. a tendency to the formation of exostoses.

Extremities.   Muscular spasm leads to tetany and occasionally paralysis.

Skin.   Ulceration and petechial haemorrhages are seen. Flat round warts are also a prominent feature.

Respiratory System.   Catarrhal involvement of mucous membranes leads to mucous discharges.

USES

The main indications for this constitutional remedy lie in the treatment of certain skeletal disorders, e.g. rickets and osteomalacia. Sessile warts on the teats and udders of heifers will benefit from treatment by this remedy. As a prophylactic against milk fever it may be combined with magnesium phosphoricum and given weekly for the last two months of pregnancy. Calcium in homoeopathic potency is the only sure way for establishing the element in the system where a deficiency exists. Young animals which need calcarea are invariably fat and slothful with slow dentition.

Calcarea Fluorica

Fluoride of Lime.   The Ø is prepared from trituration of the salt and solution in distilled water.

Crystals of this salt are found in the Haversian canals of bones. This increases the hardness of bone and in excess may result in brittleness. It also occurs in tooth enamel and in the epidermis. Affinity with all these tissues may lead to the establishment of exostoses and enlargement of superficial glands. It is in addition a powerful vascular remedy.

Eyes.   Conjunctivitis occurs and in chronic states cataract develops.

Ears. Inflammation of middle ear may extend outwards to give rise to canker in the dog and cat.

Respiratory System. Atrophy of nasal bones occurs leading in the early stages to rhinitis. Coughing is constant.

Skeletal System. Bones of the upper jaw become swollen and in extreme cases become rarefied. This extends to gums and teeth, the enamel of which becomes black and brittle. Osseous tumours may appear anywhere while gouty enlargement of joints occurs with synovitis.

Alimentary System. Induration of tongue may be seen. The changes in the gums and teeth referred to lead to loosening of teeth. The throat becomes inflamed and tonsillitis develops. Appetite is weak with flatulence and diarrhoea.

Circulatory System. The changes here are seen mainly in the venous system giving rise to engorgements and distensions with consequent oedema of various parts. Valvular disease may also occur.

Skin. The epidermis becomes thickened with the production of fistulous ulcers with raised edges and which do not heal easily.

Female Genital System. Mammary glands may show stony hard indurations.

Lymphatic System. Glands become swollen and tender to touch and later become indurated. These changes may also extend to the lymphatic vessels in severe cases.

USES

The special sphere of this remedy lies in its relation to bone and connective tissue lesions, especially exostoses and glandular swellings. Both actinomycosis and actinobacillosis of cattle should improve. Nodular tumours of the mammae in bitches come within its orbit, as also does mastitis in the cow. Given over long periods at infrequent intervals it will materially aid bone conditions such as pedal ostitis, splints, ringbone and sesamoiditis. Its action on the eye should be kept in mind in relation to its possible use in the treatment of cataract.

Calcarea Phosphorica

Phosphate of Lime.   The Ø is prepared from trituration and solution in distilled water.

This substance is prepared by adding dilute phosphorous acid to lime-water. it has an affinity with tissues which are concerned with growth and the repair of cells. Assimilation is deficient because of impaired nutrition and delayed development. Brittleness of bones may occur.

Eyes. Corneal opacities and ulcerations develop with a tendency to cataracts.

Ears. Discharge of acrid material which excoriates the ear flaps.

Alimentary System. Swelling of throat with delayed dentition. In young animals there is colicky diarrhoea after feeding.

Glandular System. Lymph gland swellings may arise in young subjects.

Urinary System. Increased output of pale urine.

Male Genital System. Swelling of testicles.

Extremities. Stiffness of muscles accompanies pain and swelling of joints. Long bones are tender to the touch.

USES

This is a remedy of special value in the treatment of many conditions of the young growing animal, e.g. rickets and milk diarrhoea. In the adult diabetes insipidus could benefit. It is not unlike calcarea carbonica in its uses but is more adapted to the lean animal of rigid fibre than to the fat sluggish patient.

Calcarea Sulphurica

Plaster of Paris. The Ø is prepared from trituration and solution in distilled water.

Suppurative processes come within the range of this substance. Mucous discharges become lumpy and thick while cystic tumours may arise.

Eyes. Ophthalmia accompanied by a thick yellow discharge.

Ears. Inflammation of middle ear with blood-stained discharge.

Alimentary System. Tonsillitis which becomes suppurative with abscess formation. Mucous diarrhoea occurs with occasionally the presence of pus. Anal abscesses develop.

Respiratory System. Purulent sputum accompanies coughing. There may be a septic pleuritis.

Skin. Wounds do not heal easily, remaining unhealthy looking and discharging pus. Sinuses and fistulas develop.

USES

Septic conditions in general call for this remedy, the chief guiding symptom being pus which has found an outlet. It is less indicated in deeper pyogenic conditions. Anal gland abscess in the dog is frequently treated with this remedy. Superficial sinuses and fistulae discharging pus will respond well.

Calendula Officinalis

Marigold.   *N.O.* Compositae.   The Ø is prepared from leaves and flowers.

   Applied locally to open wounds this tincture will be found to be one of the best healing agents. It will rapidly produce resolution of all wounds and indolent ulcers promoting healthy granulation.

   Alimentary System.   Sub-maxillary glands become swollen and the animal resents them being touched. Morning diarrhoea.

   Urinary System.   Output of urine is increased, the urine being pale and clear.

   Extremities.   Axillary lymph glands become swollen and painful.

USES

This is the chief remedy to be considered when dealing with all open wounds, being applied in a strength of 1/10 of the Ø. When dealing with jagged wounds involving damage to nerve endings it should be combined with Hypericum Ø. It is of great value in healing the gums after dental extractions rapidly reducing pain and hastening healing. As an adjunct to its local use it should be given internally when it will be found to be of value in all potencies.

Camphora

Camphor.   *N.O.* Lauraceae.   The Ø is obtained from the gum which is found in the plant.

   This plant produces a state of collapse with weakness and failing pulse. There is icy coldness of the entire body. It has a direct relationship to muscles and fascia.

   Eyes.   The animal has a fixed, staring look with dilated pupils.

   Respiratory System.   Persistent nose-bleeding and nasal discharge. Mucous material gathers in the larynx making breathing difficult.

   Alimentary System.   The jaws become clenched and salivation is copious. Diarrhoea is black and accompanies a state of collapse. Tongue and mouth are cold.

   Urinary System.   Retention of urine with strangury. Bladder becomes full with inability to expel the contents.

   Extremities.   Movement is difficult. Joints become affected, particularly the stifle. They produce a cracking sound on movement.

   Skin.   Icy coldness accompanies a dark livid appearance.

USES

Certain forms of calf scour could well benefit from this remedy, when dark stools accompany icy coldness and collapse. It is of use in shock when the pulse becomes weak and heart failure is threatened. It is of value in salmonellosis in all species.

Cannabis Sativa

American Hemp.   *N.O.* Cannabinaceae.   The Ø is prepared from the male and female flowering tops.

This plant affects particularly the urinary, sexual and respiratory spheres, conditions being accompanied by great fatigue.

Eyes.   Corneal opacities appear which progress to cataract formation.

Respiratory System.   There is a tendency to pneumonia, producing rapid breathing and palpitation.

Cardiac System.   The pericardial covering of the heart becomes inflamed.

Urinary System.   Retention of urine is accompanied by painful urging. Cystitis occurs leading to a muco-purulent discharge, possibly blood-stained.

Male Sexual System.   Balanitis and orchitis both occur.

Female Sexual System.   Tendency to abortion.

USES

This is a useful remedy in genito-urinary conditions, especially cystitis and some forms of Bright's Disease. Cataract and corneal opacities may benefit. Also inflammatory conditions of the penis, sheath and testicles.

Cantharis

Spanish Fly.   The Ø is prepared from trituration of the entire insect with subsequent dilution in alcohol.

This drug attacks particularly the urinary and sexual organs setting up a violent inflammation. The skin is also severely affected.

Eyes.   Sight becomes weak and various complaints lead to ophthalmia.

Respiratory System.   Epistaxis is a usual feature.

Alimentary System.   The tongue is covered with vesicles producing a tenacious mucus. Spasm of the throat muscles leads to difficulty in drinking. Thirst is prominent. Bloated abdomen occurs with abdominal tenderness. Gastro-enteritis is a common feature leading to peritonitis. In the dog, cat and pig there is blood-stained vomition, while dysentery occurs in all species.

Urinary System. There is severe urging to urinate, blood-stained urine coming in drops with great distress. The animal may cry out in pain. The bladder is severely affected with acute inflammation. Acute nephritis is a constant feature.

Skin. Vesicular eruptions occur with great burning and itching leading to raw patches which may become secondarily infected producing pustular lesions.

Female Genital System. Inflammation of the uterus develops as a result of extension from the bladder, particularly evident if it coincides with parturition. Swelling of vulva occurs.

USES

This is a valuable remedy in nephritis and cystitis attended by great serangury. Post-partum inflammation may require it. Eczema with the characteristic burning vesicular rash will benefit. Gastro-enteric conditions attended by severe straining and dysentery may also need this remedy. The pain and discomfort of insect bites are relieved.

Capsicum

Cayenne Pepper. *N.O.* Solanaceae. The Ø is prepared from the dried pods.

This substance affects mucous membranes and produces inflammations with a tendency to suppuration.

Ears. Swelling occurs behind the ears with signs of pain evidenced by head shaking and whimpering. Discharge of purulent material may take place.

Alimentary System. Inflammation of the gums accompanies a tenacious mucus. The throat is covered with a diptheric membrane. There may be colic with a mucoid blood-stained diarrhoea.

Urinary System. There is difficulty in passing urine which is sometimes blood-tinged.

Respiratory System. Oppression of breathing accompanied by cough.

USES

This remedy could be of use in certain forms of otitis externa. Rodent ulcer in the cat has yielded to it. Pharyngitis and septic throats could benefit. In all complaints the animal seeks warmth.

Carbo Animalis

Animal Charcoal.   The Ø is prepared from trituration and solution in distilled water.

This substance is particularly adapted to the older animal showing venous stasis of various parts.

Eyes.   Weakness of sight with dilation of pupils.

Ears.   Discharge of purulent material.

Respiratory System.   Epistaxis and fluent coryza. Dry cough which is worse at night.

Alimentary System.   Swelling of gums which are covered by purulent vesicles. Accumulation of mucus in the throat. Distress after eating. Rumbling of flatus secondary to abdominal tympany. Stools generally hard.

Urinary System.   Polyuria. The urine tends to excoriate the sheath and vulva.

Female Genital System.   Nodular tumours appear in the mammary glands.

Glandular System.   Swelling of parotid glands and of the axillary region.

Skin.   Generalised itching accompanying an erysipeloid inflammation. Soft wart-like excresences may develop.

USES

A remedy mainly for the older dog and cat, giving good results in various conditions which may affect the geriatric animal, e.g. venous stasis. Mammary growths and skin affections.

Carbo Vegetabilis

Vegetable Charcoal.   Trituration of the dried substance provides the basis of the Ø.

Various tissues of the body have a marked affinity with this substance. The circulation is particularly affected leading to lack of oxygenation with a corresponding increase of carbon dioxide in the blood and tissues. This leads to a lack of resistance to infections and to haemorrhages of dark blood which does not readily coagulate. Coldness of body surfaces ensues.

Eyes.   Agglutination of eyelids after sleep.

Respiratory System.   Nasal discharges and bleeding. Haemorrhage also takes place from the lungs. Pneumonia may develop. Yellowish expectoration is not uncommon. Asthmatic wheezing may occur in the older subject.

Alimentary System. Aphthous ulcers develop in the mouth. Abdominal discomfort sets in after eating with tympany and tenderness over the area of the stomach. Flatulent colic with rumbling of flatus occurs in severe cases.

Extremities. There is a heaviness of movement accompanied by stiffness of limbs and joints. A general lack of muscular energy is a feature.

Skin. Small haemorrhages are seen arising from superficial veins. The skin itself is cold with a disposition on the part of the animal to scratch vigorously.

Cardiac System. The pulse is small, thready and weak.

USES

This is a very useful remedy in all cases of shock and collapse from whatever cause. It is one of the stand-by remedies in flatulent colic. It should be remembered in venous pulmonary congestion and will restore warmth and strength in impending collapse. Animals exhibiting poor digestion with eructation will benefit greatly from this remedy.

Carbolicum Acidum

Phenol. The Ø is prepared from solution of the acid in rectified spirit.

Paralysis of varying degrees may result from poisoning by this acid with feeble pulse and depressed breathing due to threatened paralysis of the respiratory centre.

Alimentary System. Diphtheric lesions develop on the throat. In the dog, cat and pig dark green vomiting occurs. Flatulence and blood-stained diarrhoea follows severe enteritis.

Urinary System. Urine becomes dark brown and may contain glucose. Output is increased. Threatened uraemia.

Female Genital System. Inflammation of the uterus may occur especially after parturition.

Skin. Dermatitis is seen with a tendency to formation of ulcers.

Respiratory System. Putrid nasal discharge accompanies influenza-like weakness with coughing and dyspnoea.

Extremities. Muscle cramping affects the hind-legs, particularly below the stifle. Paretic conditions set in with stiffness of joints.

USES

Weak, debilitated and paretic conditions will benefit from this remedy. In threatened uraemia in the dog it may be needed when the urine becomes dark green-brown and oily.

Cardus Marianus

St. Mary's Thistle.   *N.O.* Compositae.   The Ø is prepared from trituration of the seeds.

The active principle of this plant acts on the liver and portal
system and on the circulation generally.

Alimentary System.   In the dog, cat and pig vomiting and
retching are first seen. The portal blood-vessels become engorged leading to swelling of liver tissue and interference with bile-flow with
consequent jaundice. Interference with the portal circulation leads to
ascites.

Urinary System.   Deep yellow or golden-coloured urine.

USES

This is a useful remedy in the treatment of many congestive and cirrhotic conditions of the liver, especially those of long-standing. Acetonaemia in the cow could well respond if other characteristic symptoms
are present while it should be remembered as a possible adjunct remedy
in canine hepatitis. Any condition showing jaundice as a prominent
symptom may improve.

Caulophyllum

Blue Cohosh.   *N.O.* Berberidaceae.   The Ø is prepared from trituration of the root.

This plant produces its main effects on the female genital system.
Small joints are also affected.

Female Genital System.   Rigidity of the os uteri is a prominent symptom, leading to difficulty at parturition. Early abortions may
occur, accompanied by fever and thirst. Retention of afterbirth is commonplace along with bleeding from the uterus.

Extremities.   Stiffness and arthritis develop in small joints,
(knee and hock) giving rise to pain and disinclination to move.

USES

This remedy revives labour pains and could be used as an alternative to
Pituitrin. It has been used successfully in ringwomb in the ewe. It will
help establish a normal pregnancy, regulating the entire gestation. Post-
partum it has proved of value in treating haemorrhage with retained
placenta. It is one of the main remedies to be considered in the treatment of pyometritis especially in those cases where the discharge is
chocolate-coloured and free flowing. It should be remembered also as a
useful remedy in some forms of small joint stiffness.

Causticum

Potassium Hydrate. This substance is prepared by the distillation of a mixture of equal parts of slaked lime and potassium bisulphate.

The main affinity is with the neuro-muscular system producing weakness and paresis of both types of muscle. Symptoms are aggravated by going from a cold atmosphere to a warm one.

Head. There is a tendency to facial paralysis. Warts also develop in the older animal.

Eyes. Inflammation of eyelids may proceed to the establishment of corneal ulcers. Degenerative lesions develop, e.g. cataract.

Ears. Both otitis media and externa are seen.

Respiratory System. Nasal ulceration leads to discharge of muco-purulent material. A dry cough occurs.

Alimentary System. Paralysis of the mouth is evidenced by inability to move the tongue properly. Bleeding from gums may occur. Abdominal bloating develops after feeding.

Urinary System. Retention of urine sets in dependent on weak bladder musculature. This may lead to cystitis.

Extremities. Paresis of single parts gives rise to various complications such as contracted tendons and stiffness of joints.

Skin. Cutaneous warts develop which bleed easily. Pruritus accompanies a pimply eruption and ulcers may arise producing a thin pus.

USES

This remedy is frequently indicated in the older subject showing early paresis, e.g. facial paralysis and rheumatic-like stiffness. Flat warts on the face of old dogs call for this remedy, and these may develop elsewhere also. It is a useful remedy in bronchitic conditions showing a harsh dry cough. It is said to have an antidotal effect in mild lead poisoning. Generalised stiffness with or without contracted tendons may benefit. It is one of the main remedies to be considered in chronic cystitis.

Ceanothus

New Jersey Tea. *N.O.* Rhamnaceae. The Ø is prepared from the fresh leaves.

This plant exerts a specific action on the spleen and is also a useful haemostat, markedly reducing the clotting time.

Respiratory System. Chronic bronchitic cough arises giving a profuse secretion of mucoid material.

Alimentary System. Inflammation and enlargement of spleen with tenderness over the liver area. Diarrhoea or dysentery may occur.

Urinary System. There is strong urging to urinate, the urine containing bile pigments.

USES

Conditions involving the spleen will probably benefit from this remedy. Its haemostatic properties should be remembered.

Chamomilla

N.O. Compositae. The Ø is prepared from the whole fresh plant.

The chief affinity of this plant is for the nervous system inducing over-excitability and hyper-sensitivity. There is extreme irritability and bad temper in suckling animals.

Eyes. Inflammation of eyelids and cornea which may assume a yellow colour.

Ears. Swelling and inflammation.

Alimentary System. Parotid and sub-maxillary glands become swollen. Abdominal tympany develops. During dentition excessive saliva and a greenish diarrhoea may be seen.

Respiratory System. Epistaxis may be accompanied by a sticky mucus.

Female Genital System. Tenderness and swelling of mammary glands. Uterine bleeding may occur, the blood being dark and clotted.

Skin. Exanthematous eruptions occur in conjunction with dentition.

USES

Its main application is as a teething remedy for pups. A variety of symptoms may arise at this time ranging from digestive upsets to involvement of the central nervous system and the remedy will bring relief in most cases. Some forms of false pregnancy have been successfully treated.

Chelidonium Majus

Greater Celandine. *N.O.* Papaveraceae. The entire plant at flowering is used in the preparation of the Ø.

A specific action on the liver is produced along with indisposition and general lethargy.

Eyes. Conjunctivitis with lachrymation. Sclerotics become yellow.

Alimentary System. The tongue is coated yellow. Inflammation of the stomach occurs with vomiting in the dog, cat and pig. The liver is constantly upset with the appearance of clay-coloured stools. Jaundice is usually present.

Urinary System. Disturbances of biliary function produces a deep yellow urine.

Extremities. Stiffness of neck muscles extending down to right shoulder area produces tenderness over the area.

Skin. Jaundice with a tendency to pustular rashes.

Respiratory System. A right-sided pneumonia develops with copious expectoration.

USES

Because of its action on the liver we should consider it in illnesses like hepatitis and even sluggishness of action where a prominent symptom is jaundice. It is useful also in certain eye conditions. Touch and movement aggravate.

Chimaphilla Umbellata

Ground Holly. *N.O.* Ericaceae. The Ø is prepared from the fresh plant in flower.

This plant produces a marked action on the kidneys and genital system of both sexes.

Eyes. Lachrymation is a constant feature while cataract may develop.

Urinary System. Urging to urinate, the urine being turbid and containing blood and mucus, and occasionally sugar.

Male Genital System. Enlargement of prostate gland occurs.

Female Genital System. Tumours of the mammary gland develop with increased secretion of milk. Later degeneration or atrophy of mammary tissue ensues.

Skin. Superficial lymphatic glands show enlargement.

USES

A useful remedy in genito-urinary conditions especially of the older dog and bitch. Prostatitis and kidney gravel will be particularly influenced.

Cicuta Virosa

Water Hemlock. *N.O.* Umbelliferae. The Ø is prepared from the fresh root when the plant flowers.

This plant exerts its main influence on the central nervous system giving rise to spasmodic affections. A characteristic feature is violence of one kind or another and an aggravation from jarring or sudden movement.

Head.   Usually turned or twisted to one side. Cerebro-spinal disorders. Balance becomes upset and there is a tendency to fall to one side. The head may bend backwards with the neck curved.

Eyes.   Dilation of pupils alternates with contraction. Eyes assume a fixed staring look.

Ears.   Mucoid discharges.

Extremities.   Spasm of muscles at base of head and on the neck throwing the head backwards. Violent jerking sets in with grinding of teeth and clenching of jaws.

Alimentary System.   Perversion of appetite with difficulty in swallowing.

Skin.   Eruptions and pustules develop which form yellow crusts. Itching is absent.

USES

Various conditions affecting the brain and spinal cord may benefit from this remedy, e.g. cerebro-cortical necrosis. It could also be indicated as an adjunct remedy in the treatment of swayback and tetanus. Post-distemper chorea in dogs has shown encouraging response. Horses and cattle are especially susceptible to poisoning by this plant.

Cimcifuga Racemosa
Actaea Racemosa

Black Snake Root.   *N.O.* Ranunculaceae.   The root provides the basis of the Ø.

There is an affinity with the nervous system and also with muscular tissues. Conditions are accompanied by restlessness.

Muscular System.   Stiffness with contraction of neck and back muscles. Pain is evident over the lumbar and sacral regions. The animal resents touch and is disinclined to move. Jerking of limbs occurs with cramping and twitching.

Nervous System.   Chorea develops in various areas, especially on pressure.

Alimentary System.   Left-sided pharyngitis occurs while diarrhoea and constipation may alternate.

Urinary System.   Large amounts of urine are passed frequently.

Female Genital System.   Ovarian conditions develop, e.g. ovaritis and salpingitis with delayed ovulation.

USES

This remedy is useful in rheumatic-like stiffness of the older dog. Disturbances of ovarian function, especially important and commonly seen in cattle, may benefit. Pyometritis in the bitch when accompanied by nervous symptoms may call for it. It is one of the remedies used to control and regulate pregnancy in animals which have previously miscarried.

Cina Maritima

Wormseed. *N.O.* Compositae. The Ø is prepared from the unexpanded flower heads.

This plant produces upsets of the digestive system due to the presence of roundworms in the intestines and stomach.

Eyes. Dilated pupils.

Ears. Itching leading to the animal pawing or kicking.

Respiratory System. Nasal irritation causing the animal to rub the nose on the ground. Spasmodic coughing occurs.

Alimentary System. Hunger develops soon after food. In the dog, cat and pig vomiting occurs immediately after eating. A bloated hard abdomen accompanies diarrhoea. Anal irritation may be seen.

Urinary System. Urine becomes turbid or milky.

Extremities. Twitching and jerking of limbs.

USES

This remedy is usually reserved for young animals showing irritability, variable appetite, grinding of teeth and possibly with accompanying fits. Santonin (a derivative of Cina) has proved useful in cataract and other eye conditions such as retinitis and choroiditis. The remedy itself is principally used as a vermifuge, all potencies being effective.

Cinchona Officinalis

Peruvian Bark. *N.O.* Rubiaceae. The Ø is prepared from the dried bark.

This plant, commonly called China, contains the alkaloid quinine as its active principle. Large doses of the bark tend to produce toxic changes, e.g. nervousness, impaired leucocyte formation, haemorrhages, fever and diarrhoea. Great weakness ensues from loss of body fluids.

Respiratory System. Epistaxis together with bleeding from the lungs. A laboured slow respiration develops.

Cardiac System. Haematomas develop from various internal haemorrhages. The heart action becomes increased with a weak thready pulse.

Extremities. Joints become swollen and painful. Muscular cramps and agues develop.

Skin. Coldness of body surface. In the horse and ox severe sweating occurs. Swelling and redness of skin with induration of lymphatic glands.

USES

This remedy should always be given when an animal is suffering from debility or weakness, particularly after loss of body-fluids, e.g. haemorrhage or prolonged diarrhoea. It is useful therefore in calf scour with other indicated remedies. Illnesses which have periodic nature tend to do well under China.

Cistus Canadensis

Rock Rose. *N.O.* Cistaceae. The Ø is prepared from tincture of the whole plant.

This plant has a strong affinity for the glandular system and to a lesser extent for the lymphatic system. Poisoned wounds and ulcerations are produced. It acts strongly on the naso-pharyngeal area.

Ears. Discharge of watery pus occurs.

Alimentary System. Gums become swollen while breath, tongue and throat feel cold. Tonsillar tissue becomes involved leading to swelling of throat glands which later become suppurative. Diarrhoea commonly sets in.

Skin. Lymph glands, especially of the neck, become enlarged and indurated.

Female Genital System. The general glandular involvement produces swelling and hardness of the mammary glands.

USES

This remedy may be of use in mild cases of Hodgkin's Disease in the dog. It will help throat conditions associated with glandular swellings with or without suppuration. Rodent ulcer in the cat has been alleviated. It should be remembered in mastitis when the udder shows persistent hard swellings, and may give good results therefore in summer mastitis.

Cocculus

Indian Cockle. *N.O.* Menispermacrae. The Ø is prepared from powdered seeds which contain an alkaloid picrotoxine. This plant produces spasmodic and paretic affections deriving from the cerebrum, not the spinal cord. Painful contractions of the limbs and trunk and a strong tendency to vomition occurs in the dog, cat and pig. This occurs as a result of prolonged movement.

Head. Paralysis of the facial nerve is occasionally seen.

Alimentary System. There is inability to open the mouth properly. Sickness in the dog and cat occurs when travelling, although this does not occur in all subjects. Paralysis of the muscles controlling swallowing occurs while distension of abdomen may arise.

USES

This is a first choice remedy for controlling travel sickness. The action on the central nervous system implies its use in some forms of epileptiform seizures and may therefore be of use in post-distemper convulsions.

Coccus Cacti

Cochineal. The Ø is prepared from the dried bodies of the female insects.

This substance has an affinity for mucous membranes producing catarrhal inflammation.

Respiratory System. Viscid mucus accumulates in the air passages leading to difficult expectoration and spasmodic coughing.

Renal System. There is urging to urinate with a diminution in the amount of urine passed. The urine is thick, deep-coloured with a reddish deposit on standing. There is general catarrhal inflammation of the urinary tract, particularly the bladder.

USES

The action of the remedy on the urinary tract suggests its main use in veterinary practice, viz. in the treatment of many of the catarrhal conditions which arise, e.g. cystitis and urethritis. It should also be remembered in chronic respiratory states leading to expectoration of tough mucus and spasmodic coughing.

Coffea Cruda

Unroasted Coffee. *N.O.* Rubiaciaea. The Ø is prepared from the raw berries of the plant.

It produces a stimulating action on all organs, increasing nervous and vascular tone. Kidneys may become inflamed and joint pains can arise. There is extreme restlessness and hypersensitivity.

Alimentary System.   Excessive hunger with slow digestion is seen along with bloating of abdomen.

Cardiac System.   A violent irregular heart beat arises with a tense pulse.

Urinary System.   Output of urine is at first increased but later there is a tendency to suppression.

USES

The Ø is useful in digestive upsets, particularly of cattle, helping to restore stomach movements and promoting digestion. Medium potencies have a sedative effect on excitable or highly strung animals. It is therefore useful in helping to calm such subjects, especially dogs at night.

Colchicum

Meadow Saffron.   *N.O.* Lilliaceae.   The Ø is prepared from the bulb procured in spring.

This plant affects muscular tissues, periosteum and synovial membranes of joints. The corm contains the alkaloid colchicine which is a cytostatic poison, capable of disturbing the rhythm of granulocytic formation in the bone marrow, producing either an increase or a decrease in the number of leucocytes. It possesses also an anti-allergic and an anti-inflammatory action which interferes with the natural recuperative power of the body. Illnesses associated with this remedy are usually acute and severe, accompanied frequently by effusions in the small joints, particularly the tarsus.

Alimentary System.   Dryness of the mouth gives way to salivation. Inflammation of the stomach develops and is accompanied by flatulence which also develops in the large intestine. The stools tend to be dysenteric, accompanied by straining. In the dog, cat and pig there is vomiting of food and bile, especially after movement.

Urinary System.   The urine is dark and scanty and in severe illness may be suppressed.

Cardiac System.   Severe palpitation occurs, the heart-beats being audible.

Extremities.   Rheumatic-like affections of the fibro-muscular system develop with twitching, producing pains which are worse from movement. Joints also become affected with pain and stiffness.

USES

In practice this remedy has a particular value in bloat of cattle when it should be repeated at frequent intervals until relief sets in. It is also a main remedy in the treatment of flatulent colic in the horse when the right lower abdomen becomes distended with gas and there is much rumbling and expulsion of flatus. Autumnal diarrhoea and dysentery also come within its range, the latter being accompanied by tympany and tenesmus. Conditions which produce inflammation and stiffness of joints may require it and also membranous colitis and dropsical states, accompanied by the passage of scanty, dark urine. One of the guiding symptoms pointing to its use is aversion to food. Conditions requiring this remedy are generally worse from movement.

Colocynthis

Bitter Cucumber.   *N.O.* Cucumbilaceae.   The Ø is prepared from the pulped fruit. It contains a glucoside-colocynthin. This plant acts as a purgative and causes violent inflammatory lesions of the gastro-intestinal tract.

Alimentary System.   Flatulent distension of the abdomen occurs. In the dog, cat and pig, vomiting takes place while in all species there is purging with severe colicky pains which are paroxysmal in type. Both onset and relief are abrupt. Diarrhoea is yellowish and forcibly expelled.

Urinary System.   The urine may be scanty and reddish-brown.

Extremities.   Stiffness of muscles is seen, especially those of the cervical region.

Skin.   A generalised itching sets in leading to shedding of epidermal scales.

USES

This is one of the main remedies for the relief of spasmodic colic in the horse. It is indicated in those forms which are accompanied by sudden onset with signs of severe pain and in the presence of a yellowish spluttery stool. The horse attempts to obtain relief by rolling and arching of the back. Relief is also obtained by movement while aggravation occurs after eating or drinking. It should be considered in any condition which produces the characteristic symptom – relief from arching of the back.

Conium Maculatum

Hemlock.   *N.O.* Umbelliferae.   The Ø is prepared from the fresh plant when in flower. The alkaloids of this plant produce a paralytic action on the nerve ganglia, having a special affinity for motor-nerve endings. This leads to stiffness and a paralysis which tends to travel upwards.

Eyes.   Excessive lachrymation occurs with corneal ulceration. Dilation of pupils is seen with paralysis of ocular muscles.

Respiratory System. There is a tendency to epistaxis with a dry, hacking cough. Muscles governing respiration may become paralysed.

Alimentary System. Loss of power arises in swallowing. Excessive abdominal bloating occurs.

Extremities. Twitchings and chorea are a regular feature. More commonly the lower limbs show paralytic weakness which shows a disposition to travel upwards.

USES

This remedy is of great importance in treating paraplegic conditions and any weakness of hind-limbs, e.g. it has given excellent results in post-distemper paralysis in dogs where ascending potencies are generally required. It has a beneficial action on small mammary tumours in the bitch where sessile growths may occur in the older subject. Some forms of lymphadenitis will benefit when the glands become hard. The general involvement of the peripheral nervous system has led to its successful use in bladder weakness of old subjects where the expulsive powers of the bladder musculature have become weakened. Its ability to produce hardness of tissue suggests its use in rodent ulcer while prostate enlargement in the dog may benefit.

Convallaria

Lily of the Valley. *N.O.* Liliaceae. The Ø is prepared from the whole plant.

The active principle of this plant has the power to increase the quality of the heart's action. This determines the main use.

Alimentary System. The tongue assumes a broad, thick appearance and is heavily coated. The region over the stomach is sensitive to the touch while signs of colic may be present.

Respiratory System. Pulmonary congestion arises consequent to the heart's action.

Renal System. There is frequent passage of small amounts of urine which has an offensive smell.

Cardiac System. A rapid and irregular pulse produces palpitation. Signs of endocarditis may be present on auscultation.

USES

This is one of the remedies which may be needed in the treatment of congestive heart conditions and alternates well with other heart remedies. In has little action on the heart muscle and should be reserved for valvular disease with or without an accompanying endocarditis. It acts well in all potencies.

Copaiva

Balsam of Peru. *N.O.* Leguminosae. The Ø is prepared from the balsam.

This substance produces a marked action on mucous membranes, especially those of the urinary and respiratory tracts, causing a catarrhal inflammation.

Renal System. Urination becomes difficult. Inflammation of the bladder occurs leading to the presence of catarrhal mucus in the urine.

Alimentary System. Intestinal flatulence is set up with production of a mucous colitis. Colicky pains accompany passage of stool which is covered with mucus.

Male Genital System. Inflammation and swelling of testicles which become tender to the touch.

Female Genital System. There is a uterine or vaginal discharge which may contain pus and blood.

Respiratory System. Catarrhal involvement of the air passages produces a muco-purulent cough.

Skin. Redness and swelling occur especially over the abdomen. Circumscribed ulcer-like patches are evident producing an itch.

USES

The action of this remedy on the urinary tract makes it a remedy of choice in the treatment of urethritis and cystitis where the characteristic mucous deposits occur. Bitches which develop pyometra may require it if there are accompanying urinary symptoms. Its action on the skin suggests its possible use in eczema.

Crataegus

Hawthorn. *N.O.* Rosaceae. The Ø is prepared from the ripe fruit.

The active principle of this plant produces a reduction in blood-pressure and brings about difficulty in breathing. It acts on the heart muscle causing an increase in the number and quality of contractions.

Cardiac System. Myocarditis occurs with failing compensation. Irregularities of action bring about a state of anaemia with oedema of dependent parts, and in severe cases generalised anasarca.

Urinary System. There is a tendency towards the production of diabetic urine which may also contain excess albumen.

Skin. Generalised eruptions occur on most species. Horses may show excessive sweating.

USES

The specific action of the remedy on heart muscle makes it particularly useful in the treatment of arrhythmic heart conditions, especially in the older dog. It has little or no action on the linings of auricles or ventricles.

Crocus Sativus

Saffron. *N.O.* Iridaceae. The Ø is prepared from the fresh young shoots.

This plant is associated with haemorrhagic conditions where the blood becomes stringy and assumes a dark appearance. Muscular twitchings also occur.

Eyes. There is enlargement of pupils which react slowly to stimuli. Aversion to light is common with a tendency to the later development of glaucoma. Eyelids have a drooping appearance.

Respiratory System. Nasal bleeding takes place with the characteristic dark stringy blood which clots quickly. A wheezy cough may be present.

Alimentary System. Stagnation of the portal circulation leads to digestive upsets with an accompanying constipation.

Female Genital System. Bleeding from the uterus takes place. In the pregrant animal this may lead to abortion.

Extremities. Spasmodic contraction of muscles occurs together with twitching. This is usually confined to single areas and is rarely generalised. The legs become weak and there is difficulty in rising.

USES

Haemorrhages of the type referred to are the main indication for this remedy. It is useful in abortion which is attended by the passage of dark stringy clotted blood. Digestive upsets dependent on sluggish portal activity will also benefit.

Crotalus Horridus

Rattlesnake Venom. The Ø is prepared from a solution of the venom in glycerine.

The venom of this snake produces sepsis, haemorrhages and jaundice with decomposition of blood.

Eyes. The generalised jaundiced state produces a yellow colour of the sclerotics. Intra-ocular haemorrhages occur.

Respiratory System. There is nasal bleeding of black blood which fails to coagulate. Bleeding may also take place from the lungs.

Alimentary System. The tongue becomes red and swollen. Vomiting of blood takes place in the dog, cat and pig. Abdominal distension occurs with pain over the region of the liver. Rectal bleeding occurs, the blood being fluid and dark. Stools generally are dysenteric. Haemolytic jaundice is a more or less constant feature.

Female Genital System. Vaginal or uterine bleeding takes place.

Urinary System. Nephritis is accompanied by albuminuria with casts in dark bloody urine.

Cardiac System. The heart action becomes feeble with a weak thready pulse. Air hunger is evident.

Skin. Swelling with capillary bleeding takes place. Yellowish discolouration is common with the production of putrid ulcers. Wounds remain unhealthy while the skin remains dry and cold.

Lymphatic System. Generalised swelling of lymph glands and vessels.

USES

The marked action of this poison on the vascular system makes it a valuable remedy in the treatment of many septic states which show also circulatory involvement, e.g. puerperal fever and wound infections. Septic conditions are accompanied by oozing of blood from any body orifice and are usually attended by jaundice. Warfarin poisoning has been successfully treated with frequent doses of high potencies. It could prove useful in controlling the haemorrhages associated with clover poisoning. Aural haematoma in the dog and cat may be helped post-operatively in controlling the tendency to further haemorrhage. Purpura haemorrhagica should be helped as should also post-partum bleeding when the blood is dark and fluid.

Croton Tiglium

Croton Oil Seed. *N.O.* Euphorbiaceae. The Ø is prepared from the seeds which contain the oil.

This oil produces violent evacuations of the bowel and skin eruptions causing inflammation with a tendency to vesicle formation.

Eyes. Pustules develop on the cornea. Eruptions occur around the eyelids producing a raw appearance.

Alimentary System. Copious watery stools occur which are usually forcibly expelled with much urging. A gurgling sound is heard in the intestines.

Urinary System. There is production of dark orange-coloured urine which becomes turbid and greasy when passed at night. During daylight the urine is pale with a white sediment.

Skin. Vesicular eruptions occur especially on the face and genital region. These are attended by intense itching.

USES

This is one of the many useful remedies for controlling diarrhoea which is accompanied by great urging, the stool being watery. Some forms of coli-bacillosis in calves and piglets may benefit. It is also a valuable remedy in the control of vesicular eczematous eruptions.

Cubeba

Cubebs. *N.O.* Piperaceae. The Ø is prepared from the dried unripe fruit.

This plant exerts its action chiefly on the mucous membranes of the urinary tract.

Urinary System. Frequent urination occurs along with inflammation of the urethra which is the underlying cause. This is seen more often in the female. Blood appears in the urine as a secondary complication. The bladder is also affected producing cystitis. In the male there may be prostatitis.

USES

Its use is almost wholly confined to the treatment of affections of the urinary system, principally urethritis and cystitis.

Cuprum Metallicum

Copper. The Ø is prepared from trituration of the metal.

The symptoms produced by this metal are characterised by violence. Paroxysms of cramps come and go and can be initiated by fright. They generally appear suddenly.

Eyes. May be turned upwards and are fixed and staring.

Alimentary System. Jaws become contracted with a tendency to foaming at the mouth. Protrusion and retraction of the tongue alternate. In the dog and cat and pig, vomiting occurs while there is colic and diarrhoea in all species.

Cardiac System. There is usually a slow pulse.

Extremities. Muscular cramps and stiffness develop with chronic spasms producing jerking and twitching.

Central Nervous System. Fits and convulsions can occur of an epileptic nature. The head may be drawn to one side.

USES

Muscular cramp is a common condition which may find relief from this remedy, e.g. in greyhounds. It is also of service in the treatment of copper deficiency in cattle. Oesophageal spasm may also benefit. Occasional doses have been found to benefit racing animals, e.g. thoroughbreds and hunters which may suffer from muscular cramping in various forms.

Curare

Arrow Poison. *N.O.* Loganiaceae. The Ø is prepared from dilution of the poison in alcohol.

This poison produces muscular paralysis without impairing sensation or consciousness. Reflex action is diminished and a state of motor paralysis sets in. It decreases the output of adrenalin and brings about a state of nervous debility.

Alimentary System. In the mouth buccal and facial paralysis occur. The tongue may be drawn to one side, frequently the right.

Respiratory System. Difficult breathing may be so severe as to threaten respiration entirely.

Extremities. Paresis of muscles is preceded by trembling of limbs.

Skin. Boils appear accompanied by itching. There is a tendency to cutaneous haemorrhage in the region of these eruptions.

USES

Some forms of post-distemper paralysis may be helped by this remedy, notably those in which the dog shows no involvement of the central nervous system. Paralysis of single parts, e.g. radial, may benefit. Post-influenzal debility and weakness in the horse may also show improvement.

Digitalis

Foxglove.   *N.O.* Scrophulariaceae.   The Ø is prepared from the leaves.

The active principle of the foxglove causes a marked reduction in the heart's action, the pulse becoming weak and irregular.

Alimentary System.   Salivation occurs and in the dog, cat and pig there may be vomiting. The liver becomes enlarged and ascites is usually present.

Renal System.   Frequent urging to urinate is seen, the urine being dark and scanty. Inflammation of the urethra is a common sequel.

Respiratory System.   Inflammation of the bronchial mucous membrane results in oppressive breathing.

Cardiac System.   Irregular heart beat arises and mitral valve incompetence may occur. Dilation of the heart leads eventually to hypertrophy of the heart muscle.

Extremities.   As a result of the slowing down of the circulation oedema of dependent parts sets in, e.g. ascites in the smaller animals and swelling of the legs and brisket of horses and cattle.

USES

A commonly used remedy in heart affections of the older dog especially. It helps regulate the beat and produces a stable pulse. By increasing the output of the heart when used in low potencies it aids valvular function. This in turn will affect the output of urine and help reduce oedema.

Drosera

Sundew.   *N.O.* Droseraceae.   The Ø is prepared from tincture of the fresh plant.

The lymphatics, pleural and synovial membranes are all affected by this plant. The laryngeal area is also subject to inflammatory processes, any stimulus producing a hypersensitive reaction.

Respiratory System.   Spasmodic dry cough is a fairly constant symptom, paroxyms following each other quickly. The pleurae become involved producing a rapid short breath.

USES

In veterinary practice its use is restricted to pulmonary and laryngeal affections. Principally pleurisy with dry paroxysmal cough. Some types of pneumonia and upper tracheitis. It has given good results in virus pneumonia of calves. Its association with tuberculosis has little relevance today but we should remember its ability to absorb scar tissue and in this connection it may be grouped along with Silicea and Graphites.

Dulcamara

Woody Nightshade. *N.O.* Solanaceae. The Ø is prepared from fresh leaves before flowering.

This plant belongs to the same family as Belladonna, Hyoscyamus and Stramonium. Tissue affinities are with mucous membranes, muscles, glands and kidneys, producing inflammatory changes and interstitial haemorrhages.

Eyes. A watery discharge occurs, leading to catarrhal ophthalmia.

Alimentary System. A sticky saliva appears with ulceration of mouth. Scraping of the throat occurs. In the dog, cat and pig, mucous vomiting takes place while colic and diarrhoea are seen in all species. Stools tend to be yellowish or greenish-tinged.

Lymphatic System. In wet weather there is a tendency to swelling of the lymph glands.

Renal System. Any exposure to chill produces profuse urination, the urine being turbid due to the presence of mucus.

Respiratory System. Accumulation of mucus leads to a loose rattling cough and nasal discharge.

Extremities. Paralysis occurs in various parts and is accompanied by icy coldness of affected areas. Muscular spasm may be present.

Skin. Warty excrescences develop while vesicular eruptions lead to itching.

USES

This remedy should benefit those conditions which arise as a result of exposure to wet and cold, especially when damp evenings follow a warm, dry day. Such conditions commonly occur in autumn and diarrhoea occurring then may benefit. Symptoms calling for this remedy tend to alternate with one another, e.g. skin eruptions with muscular stiffness. It has proved useful in the treatment of ringworm and has a beneficial action on large, sessile warts. Equine colic arising from exposure to cold and damp will be relieved. The action on the kidney suggests that it may be beneficial in acute interstitial nephritis.

Echinacea

Rudbeckia. *N.O.* Compositae. The Ø is prepared from the whole fresh plant.

Acute toxaemias with septic involvement of various tissues come within the sphere of action of this plant.

Alimentary System. Ulceration of tongue and gums takes place with associated bleeding. The tonsillar tissue becomes dark and swollen.

Renal System. Scanty albuminous urine, dependent on nephritis.

Female Genital System. Puerperal fever with sepsis may arise. Discharges are usually scanty leading to toxaemia.

Skin. Recurrent boils and pimply swellings are common. Neglected cases may lead to gangrene.

Lymphatic System. Enlarged lymph glands appear accompanying a septic lymphangitis.

USES

This is a valuable remedy in post-partum discharges and conditions where sepsis is evident. It is particularly useful in the bitch and mare. Generalised toxaemic states having their origin in infected bites or stings will benefit. This remedy acts best in low potency, e.g 3x.

Elaps Corallinus

Coral Snake. The venom is triturated with sugar of milk to provide the basis for the preparation of potencies.

The action of this venom is similar in general to snake poisons as a whole, but discharges tend to be more black than usual.

Eyes. There is strong aversion to light.

Ears. Accumulation of hard wax accompanies a greenish discharge which tends to darken. Severe itching.

Alimentary System. The throat is chiefly affected. Dry crusts form in the pharyngeal region.

Respiratory System. Haemorrhage takes place from the lungs, the blood being dark and remaining fluid.

Skin. Severe itching is usual with a tendency to peeling. Vesicular eruptions occur on the feet.

Extremities. Lymphangitis may arise giving the legs a swollen appearance.

USES

Septic conditions with oozing of dark fluid blood come within the sphere of action of this remedy as with other snake venoms, but conditions are usually less severe when Elaps is called for. Some forms of ear canker may benefit. Its symptomatology suggests that it may be of use in the early stages of canine viral hepatitis, and also in equine lymphangitis – so-called 'Monday Morning Disease'.

Elaterium

Squirting Cucumber. *N.O.* Cucurbitaceae. The Ø is prepared from the unripe fruit.

As with Dulcamara the effects of this poison are frequently seen after exposure to damp. The digestive and cutaneous areas are mainly affected.

Alimentary System. In the dog, cat and pig, vomiting occurs with generalised weakness. In all species there is a copious watery diarrhoea of a frothy consistency and greenish tinge. Characteristic of this diarrhoea is its explosive nature.

Skin. Oedema of subcutaneous tissues accompanies uritcarial swellings.

Extremities. Nodules arise on various joints.

USES

This remedy is chiefly used to combat diarrhoea of an explosive or gushing nature and also to treat angio-neurotic conditions in the skin.

Erigeron

Fleabane. *N.O.* Compositae. The Ø is prepared from the whole plant when in bloom.

The action of this plant is associated with haemorrhages from various parts, principally from bladder and uterus.

Renal System. There is urging to urinate, the urine containing blood.

Female Genital System. Discharge of bright red blood occurs from the uterus. During pregnancy there is a tendency to prolapse.

USES

This should be remembered as one of the remedies which is useful in controlling haemorrhage, especially from the uterus. Some forms of nephritis will benefit and it could be given prophylactically to the bitch during pregnancy to help prevent prolapse.

Equisetum

Scouring Rush. *N.O.* Equisetaceae. The Ø is prepared from the fresh plant.

The principal action of this substance is on the bladder, producing a severe urging to urinate.

Renal System. The urine contains albumen and casts as a result of inflammation set up on the mucous membrane of kidney tubules and bladder. There may be difficulty in passing urine especially in the female during pregnancy.

USES

This is a prominent urinary remedy being helpful in cystitis and nephritis. It is especially valuable in incontinent, elderly subjects.

Eserinum

Eserine. Physostigmine. The Ø is prepared from solution in alcohol.

This remedy stimulates the autonomic nervous system producing contractions of smooth muscle.

Eyes. Pupils severely contracted. Blepharospasm.
Alimentary System. Salivation. Vomiting in dog and cat.
Cardiac System. Pulse small and thready.
Skin. Profuse sweating.

USES

Could be a useful remedy in feverish conditions associated with profuse sweating. Also in glaucoma. Vomiting may be controlled, other symptoms agreeing.

Eucalyptus

Blue Gum Tree. *N.O.* Myrtaceae. The Ø is prepared from the fresh leaves.

Catarrhal inflammations and intestinal disturbances are associated
with this plant.

Respiratory System. Chronic catarrhal and purulent discharges take place from the nose. Coughing produces expectoration of
muco-purulent material.

Alimentary System. There is excessive production of gas
leading to tympany. Digestion is weak and the region over the spleen
feels hard. Dysentery or diarrhoea may be present with straining.

Renal System. Acute nephritis develops with blood appearing
in the urine. Pyelonephritis may supervene.

Skin. Herpetic eruptions appear with ulcers which are slow to
heal.

USES

Nephritic conditions in general are helped by this remedy, especially
pyelonephritis in cattle. Rumenal bloat may also respond. Indefinite
digestive conditions with or without splenic involvement also suggest its
use, e.g. acetonaemia.

Euonymus Europaeae

Spindle Tree.   *N.O.* Celastraceae.   The Ø is prepared from a trituration of the dried seeds.

This plant, together with other species of Euonymus, has an affinity with the liver and kidney producing disturbance of liver metabolism and catarrhal inflammations of the urinary tract.

Alimentary System. Flatulent colic develops with alternate
diarrhoea and constipation. The mouth remains dry with attendant
thirst. Congestive states of the liver mix with impairment of the portal
circulation.

Renal System. The biliary congestion gives rise to albuminuria
and the appearance of casts and acid deposits in the urine which is
scanty and highly coloured.

Extremities. Disturbance of kidney function produces weakness and tenderness over the lumbar region.

USES

This is a useful remedy for sluggish conditions of liver and kidney seen
principally by the appearance of the urine. Such conditions accompanying flatulent colic in the horse suggests its use in preference to Colchicum or Colocynthis.

Eupatorium Perfoliatum

Thoroughwort. *N.O.* Compositae. The Ø is prepared from the whole plant.

Bronchial mucous membranes are affected by this plant. It also has a tissue affinity with stomach and liver.

Alimentary System. In the dog, cat and pig, bilious vomiting occurs. In all species diarrhoea is common, the stool being greenish. This may alternate with constipation, producing a clay-coloured stool.

Respiratory System. Bronchial coughing leads to the expectoration of muco-purulent material. Nasal discharges also occur.

Extremities. Joints in general are affected, dropsical swellings giving a puffy appearance.

USES

Infections which involve stomach and intestines together with bronchial involvement come within the sphere of action of this remedy, e.g. it will be of use in Equine Influenza and cat 'flu. Also some forms of Canine Distemper may benefit. The action on the joints suggests its possible use in synovitis and windgalls.

Eupatorium Purpureum

Gravel Root. *N.O.* Compositae. The Ø is prepared from the root.

There is a tissue affinity with the uro-genital systems of both male and female.

Renal System. The animal exhibits pain and tenderness over the kidney region. The bladder is affected, causing cystitis with blood-stained urine. Albuminuria occurs also.

Male Genital System. The prostate gland is principally affected, producing swelling with inability to express urine, and straining at stool.

Female Genital System. Inflammation of ovaries occurs together with a tendency to miscarriage.

Extremities. Stiffness over the loins and sacral region makes it difficult for the animal to rise. There is resentment on pressure over the loins and lower back.

USES

Uro-genital conditions in general may be alleviated by the use of this remedy, e.g. prostate enlargement in old dogs and renal dropsy in all species. Irregularities of the oestrus cycle in mares and cows dependent on ovarian malfunction may benefit. It could also be of use in bladder affections.

Euphorbium

Spurge Gum. *N.O.* Euphorbiaceae. The Ø is prepared from the resin extracted from the lower Euphorbia.

This substance is an irritant to the skin and mucous membranes.

Eyes. Agglutination of eyelids is a constant feature.

Alimentary System. Excessive salivation and hunger develop. Flatulence is common with signs of colic and fermented stools which tend to be clay-coloured.

Respiratory System. Nasal discharges are seen with spasmodic dry cough.

Extremities. Weakness and paresis of leg muscles sets in. The hip-joints and sacral region are tender to the touch.

Skin. Erysipiloid eruptions take place especially on the head and face. These develop into yellow blisters which finally become ulcers, which are slow to heal.

USES

This is a useful remedy in some forms of eczema showing the typical symptoms. It could have a place in the treatment of flatulent colic in the horse and in paretic or rheumatoid conditions of the older dog.

Euphrasia

Eyebright. *N.O.* Scrophulariaceae. The Ø is prepared from the whole plant.

The active principle of this plant acts mainly on the conjunctival mucous membrane producing lachrymation.

Eyes. Catarrhal conjunctivitis develops producing acrid discharges.

Respiratory System. Nasal discharges of mucous material.

Alimentary System. In the dog and cat there may be occasional vomiting. In all species a tendency to diarrhoea occurs.

USES

This is one of the most useful remedies in the treatment of a variety of eye conditions, principally conjunctivitis and corneal ulceration. It may prove useful as an adjunct remedy in the treatment of cat 'flu. Internal medication should be supplemented by its use externally as lotion diluted 1/10.

Ferrum Metallicum

Iron.   The Ø is prepared from a trituration of the metal and its carbonate.

This remedy is best adapted to young anaemic subjects.

Alimentary System.   Food is regurgitated or vomited immediately on taking it. Abdominal flatulence occurs.

Respiratory System.   Bleeding from lungs takes place along with expectoration of mucous material.

USES

It is mainly used in anaemic conditions. Gastric disorders with regurgitation of half-digested contents come within its sphere of action. In this connection it may prove useful in treating bovine actinobacillosis affecting the stomachs. Loss of appetite may alternate with ravenous hunger. It could prove effective in the control of flatulent diarrhoea and in round-worm infestations of puppies and kittens. It has a relaxing effect on certain organs and tissues and may be beneficial in rectal or vaginal prolapse. In haemorrhagic conditions the blood contains dark clots and coagulates easily.

Ferrum Phosphoricum

Iron Phosphate.   The Ø is prepared from a trituration of the salt.

Febrile conditions in general are associated with this substance.

Eyes.   Inflammation of eyelids gives a red appearance.

Ears.   Acute inflammation of various ear structures develops. In severe long-standing cases this leads to suppuration.

Respiratory System.   Nasal bleeding is a common occurrence as is also haemorrhage from the lungs resulting from congestion.

Alimentary System.   The mouth has a red appearance with ulceration of the throat.

Extremities.   Muscular stiffness develops. Joints may become swollen.

USES

This remedy is frequently indicated in the early stages of inflammatory conditions which develop less rapidly than those calling for Aconitum. Throat involvement is frequently the key to its selection. Haemorrhages arising from an active hyperaemia come within its range and are accompanied by a soft full pulse (the reverse of Aconitum). Brain and pulmonary congestions with typical haemorrhages will usually benefit, e.g. mild encephalitis or meningitis. It could prove of value in heatstroke.

Ferrum Picricum

Picrate of Iron.　　The Ø is prepared from trituration.

The skin and the renal system are affected by this salt and it also has a slight effect on the male genital system.

Skin.　　Various types of epithelial growths develop, the majority having a warty appearance.

Renal System.　　There is frequent passage of urine at night. Cystitis may develop leading to difficulty in passing urine.

Male Genital System.　　Enlargement of the prostate gland may arise.

USES

This remedy could be of use in prostatitis of the older dog. Any accompanying cystitis should benefit. The action on the skin suggests its use as one of the remedies to be considered in the treatment of warts and other benign growths.

Ficus Religiosa

Pakur.　*N.O.* Moraceae.　The Ø is prepared from the juice of the fresh leaves.

Haemorrhages of various sorts are associated with the toxic effects of this plant.

Alimentary System.　　In the dog, cat and pig vomiting of bright red blood may be seen. Tenderness over the stomach region suggests an underlying gastritis.

Respiratory System.　　Haemorrhages take place from the lungs accompanied by coughing. Breathing becomes laboured.

Cardiac System.　　A weak thready pulse develops.

Renal System.　　The general tendency to haemorrhage causes blood to appear in the urine.

USES

Any condition which produces haemorrhage of bright red blood may indicate the need for this remedy, e.g. idiopathic nose bleeding and haematuria. It could be of value in coccidiosis in calves but generally respiratory rather than digestive upsets determine its use. It has been used successfully also in uterine haemorrhage.

Flor de Piedra

Lophophytum.　The Ø is prepared from the root.

This plant which grows on the roots of certain South American trees has an affinity with the thyroid gland.

Skin.　Severe itching develops.

Glandular System.　The thyroid gland is principally affected, functional changes being caused. This in turn leads to an action on the heart.

Alimentary System.　Functional disturbances also occur in the liver and gall-bladder leading to interference with the flow of bile. There may be an accompanying hepatitis.

USES

This remedy will be of use in the treatment of thyroid conditions especially in the dog. It has also given good results in pancreatitis. Cardiac conditions associated with thyroid disturbance will benefit indirectly when that gland is treated for malfunction. Lower potencies are indicated in liver conditions while higher potencies are needed for treating thyroid conditions.

Fluoricum Acidum

Hydrofluoric Acid.　This substance is prepared by distilling calcium fluoride with sulphuric acid. The Ø is prepared from the resulting powder after trituration.

The acid acts on deeper seated tissues producing ulcerative and destructive lesions.

Ears.　Ulceration of inner ear with discharges of acrid material. Bony growths tend to appear on cartilages.

Eyes.　The lachrymal duct frequently develops a fistula.

Respiratory System.　Ulceration of the nasal septum produces a chronic discharge. Fluid gathers in the pleural cavity making breathing difficult.

Alimentary System. Dental fistula develops accompanied by blood-stained saliva. The bones and teeth of the upper jaw show necroses. The throat becomes ulcerated and there is desire for cold water. Warm drinks may bring on bouts of diarrhoea. The region over the liver becomes tender.

Renal System. The urine becomes scanty and dark. If dropsical states develop an increase in urination may occur.

Extremities. Inflammation of joints may be seen especially on the toes and nail beds.

USES

This remedy has proved useful in some forms of nephritis, especially in the older animal exhibiting signs of degenerative changes. It may be of value in Fog Fever in cattle and also in some form of ear canker in the dog and cat. Bone necroses of the upper jaw as in actinomyosis should benefit as also may dental fistula.

Fragaria Vesca

Wild Strawberry.   *N.O.* Rosaceae.   The Ø is prepared from the ripe fruit.

This plant has an affinity with the digestive system and the skin.

Alimentary System. Deposition of tartar on the teeth may be excessive. The tongue becomes swollen and red.

Skin. Urticaria wheals develop with erysipeloid swelling and petechial haemorrhage.

Female Genital System. The action on the mammary gland has an inhibitory effect on the formation of milk.

USES

The remedy will help prevent excessive deposition of tartar and should be given at regular intervals to dogs and cats after they have reached two years old. It may help establish a normal flow of milk in nursing animals if there is a deficiency.

Gelsemium Sempervirens

Yellow Jasmine. *N.O.* Loganiaceae. The Ø is prepared from the bark of the root.

The affinity with the nervous system is a characteristic of this plant producing varying degrees of motor paralysis.

Eyes. Drooping of eyelids occurs. Contraction and twitching of eye muscles is seen.

Alimentary System. Tonsillitis may arise. Weakness of throat muscles makes swallowing difficult.

Renal System. Profuse clear watery urine is the usual pattern. Expulsion of urine is difficult due to paresis of the bladder muscles.

Respiratory System. Breathing becomes slow and laboured.

Cardiac System. The pulse is slow and weak.

Extremities. Loss of power occurs in muscles, causing trembling and weakness of limbs. Incoordination of movement then arises.

USES

This remedy has aided recovery in cases of hypomagnesaemia in cattle and sheep, aiding restoration of normal movement after injection of the usual mixtures. Its use in this connection makes relapse less likely. Equine influenza has benefited and also radial paralysis as well as facial nerve weakness. Conditions which call for its use are usually attended by weakness and muscle tremors. In the mental sphere it can cause an anticipatory fear and this observation has led to its successful use in nervous animals prior to showing or racing. Roaring in horses has shown alleviation under the influence of this remedy.

Graphites

Black Lead. The Ø is prepared from trituration of fine black lead.

This form of carbon has an affinity with nails and skin. Eruptions are commonplace and the action on connective tissue tends to produce fibrotic conditions associated with malnutrition.

Eyes. Chronic conditions such as inflamed eyelids are accompanied by discharges which tend to agglutinate the eyelids.

Ears. Chronic thin excoriating discharges accompany a sticky eczema behind the ears.

Skin. Loss of hair or fur is commonly encountered. Purply moist eruptions ooze a sticky discharge. Abrasions develop into ulcers which tend to suppurate.

Alimentary System. Blisters may appear on the tongue. Constipation is usually present, stools being covered with mucus. There may be hepatitis.

Lymphatic and Glandular Systems. Cervical lymph glands become swollen while tumours develop in the mammary gland.

USES

This remedy is particularly useful in small animal practice for the particular kind of eczema which shows the characteristic moist sticky discharges. It is useful in the treatment of certain types of interdigital cyst, particularly those showing moist swellings. Favourite sites for eczema in connection with Graphites are the bends of the joints and behind the ears. Scar tissues may show resolution especially after abscess formation. Over-fed obese animals with sticky crust-laden eyelids are generally good subjects for this remedy.

Gunpowder

Black Gunpowder.   The Ø is prepared from trituration.

This substance has proved its efficacy in the treatment of various conditions of a septic or toxic nature, e.g. abscesses, blood-poisoning and infected wounds.

Hamamelis Virginica

Witch Hazel. *N.O.* Hamamelidaceae. The Ø is prepared from the fresh bark of twigs and root.

This plant has an affinity with the venous circulation, producing congestions and haemorrhages. The action on the veins is one of relaxation with consequent engorgement.

Eyes. Bloodshot appearance due to congestion of vessels.

Respiratory System. Dark non-coagulable blood comes from nose and lungs.

Alimentary System. Varicose appearance of throat veins and tonsillar tissue due to engorgement of vessels.

Renal System. There may be blood in the urine.

Skin. Purpura-like haemorrhages appear along with traumatic lesions.

USES

Any condition showing venous congestion and passive haemorrhage from veins should show improvement under this remedy. Epistaxis and haemoptysis of venous origin as sometimes occur in racing animals has been successfully treated. Purpura-like conditions will also respond. It hastens absorption of blood from intra-ocular haemorrhage.

Hecla Lava

Volcanic Ash. The Ø is prepared from trituration of the ash.

Present in this ash are the substances which accompany lava formation viz. alumina, lime and Silica. Lymphoid tissue and the skeletal system are areas which show the greatest affinity with this substance.

Skeletal System. The bony area which is mainly affected is the upper jaw, injuries to which may lead to exostoses or tumour formation.

Lymphatic System. Lymph glands become hard and inflamed, especially those of the neck.

USES

This remedy is useful in the treatment of exostoses or tumours of the facial bones, or caries arising from dental disease. It has been used successfully in the treatment of actinomycosis of the mandible in cattle. It may be used with advantage in rhinitis and in bone necroses generally.

Helleborus Niger

Christmas Rose. *N.O.* Ranunculaceae. The Ø is prepared from the juice of the fresh root.

The affinity of this plant is with the central nervous system and the alimentary canal. To a lesser extent the kidneys are involved.

Central Nervous System. Vertigo-like movements arise together with convulsions arising possibly from meningitis.

Alimentary System. Vomiting occurs in the dog, cat and pig. In all species there is salivation and purging with dysenteric stools. Swallowing is difficult and abdominal dropsy is present.

Cardiac System. The heart's action is slowed with a thready pulse developing. Output of blood is decreased.

Renal System. Interference with kidney function leads to scanty urine which is dark with a reddish-brown sediment.

Extremities. There is usually retraction of the head and twitching of muscles.

USES

This remedy may be of use in controlling affections of the brain and spinal cord which lead to a lack of response to external stimuli. It could have a place in the treatment of cerebro-cortical necrosis of sheep and cattle and also in the nervous sequelae of canine distemper. Its action on the heart suggests its use as a cardiac remedy, other symptoms being equal.

Helonias Dioica

Unicorn Root. *N.O.* Melanthaceae. The Ø is prepared from the root.

The active principle of this plant affects mainly the lumbo-sacral region.

Renal System. Output of urine is greatly increased. The urine has a low specific gravity and may at times be albuminous.

Female Genital System. Mammary glands become swollen. Miscarriage may occur in the gravid uterus.

Back and Loins. There is marked tenderness over the lumbo-sacral region.

USES

This remedy has a place in the treatment of lumbo-sacral conditions showing weakness especially in the female. Animals which have shown previous miscarriages may benefit as also will those which have a history of sterility. In the dog diabetes insipidus is likely to benefit. The action on the mammary gland suggests that it could be of value in the control of false pregnancy. Uterine conditions in general will react favourably.

Hepar Sulphuris Calcareum

Calcium Sulphide.   The Ø is prepared from the ash resulting from burning calcium carbonate and sulphur and after trituration, dissolved in alchohol.

This substance is associated with suppurative processes producing conditions which are extremely sensitive to touch. It causes catarrhal and purulent inflammation of mucous membranes in general.

Eyes.   Purulent conjunctivitis. Corneal ulcer develops with suppurative iritis.

Ears.   Otitis media and externa leading to blood-stained and evil-smelling discharge.

Respiratory System.   Purulent pneumonia and empyema.

Alimentary System.   Suppurative processes develop in the throat and soft palate. Liver abscess may occur leading to abdominal tympany. Chronic abdominal affections are commonplace.

Lymphatic System.   Rapid suppuration follows involvement of the disease process in the lymph glands. These become infected from neighbouring purulent conditions.

Skin.   Pustular involvement leads to the development of boils and suppurative processes generally. Abscesses, ulcers and eczematous conditions are all encountered and are characterised by extreme sensitivity.

USES

The numerous conditions which this remedy will aid are all characterised by suppuration at some stage, and all have the low pain threshold. Even cold air blowing on a lesion will produce pain. Conditions frequently met with and which should show response to treatment include interdigital cysts, ear canker, Summer mastitis and chronic abscess formation. In the horse fistulous withers and various forms of bursitis may respond well. Lower potencies of this remedy e.g. 1x – 3x will promote suppuration, while higher ones, e.g. 200c – 1m will abort the suppurative process.

Hydrangea Arborescens

N.O. Hydrangeaceae.   The Ø is prepared from fresh leaves and young shoots.

This plant exerts a strong influence on the urinary system especially on the bladder where it helps dissolve gravel. The prostate gland is also affected.

USES

Useful in the control of various forms of lithiasis and in enlarged prostate of old dogs. It has been found useful also in some cases of diabetes insipidus.

Hydrastis Canadensis

Golden Seal.   *N.O.* Ranunculaceae.   The Ø is prepared from the fresh root.

Mucous membranes are affected by the plant, a catarrhal inflammation being established. Secretions are generally thick and become yellow or purulent due to secondary infection.

Ears.   A muco-purulent discharge develops.

Respiratory System.   Thick purulent nasal discharge occurs with a tendency to ulceration of the septum. A dry cough leading to bronchial catarrh when the cough becomes moist.

Alimentary System.   Inflammation of the throat is seen showing white spots. Gastritis leads to a weak digestive process. There is tenderness over the liver with jaundice and dry stools.

Extremities.   Stiffness and pain develop over the lumbar region.

Skin.   Ulceration with variola-like eruptions.

Female Genital System.   Catarrhal and purulent discharges occur from the womb. These may at times be blood-stained while whole blood may be passed independently of other discharge. Mammary tumours develop which are hard and irregular in outline.

USES

Catarrhal conditions in general come within the scope of this remedy. It has been used successfully in the treatment of pyometritis. Some forms of cat 'flu will benefit and also rhinitis of long-standing. Its early use in treating mammary tumour will prevent development of the growth and have a beneficial effect generally on the mammary gland. It should be remembered also in connection with liver and digestive disorders resulting in jaundice and light coloured stools.

Hydrocyanicum Acidum

Hydrocyanic Acid. The Ø is prepared from solutions of the gas in water.

This substance produces various epileptic and convulsive states with generalised collapse following respiratory failure.

Head. Jaws clenched tight.

Alimentary System. Frothing at mouth. Tongue cold and cyanosed. Colicky pains.

Respiratory System. Suffocative breathing and coughing. Venous congestion of lungs.

Cardiac System. Pulse weak and irregular.

USES

This remedy has been used successfully in some forms of equine colic where the patient shows symptoms of collapse. It could also be of use in threatened respiratory failure with the typical cyanosed appearance of visible mucous membranes.

Hyoscyamus Niger

Henbane. *N.O.* Solanaceae. The Ø is prepared from the fresh plant.

The active principle of this plant disturbs the central nervous system producing symptoms of excitement and mania.

Head. Involvement of the brain leads to severe head shaking and possibly unconsiousness.

Eyes. The pupils of the eyes are dilated and fixed with spasmodic closing of the lids.

Alimentary System. The tongue is red and dry, being protruded with difficulty. There may be foaming of the mouth with sordes on the teeth. Drooping of the lower jaw produces an inability to swallow. In the dog, cat and pig there is vomiting with convulsions. Bleeding takes place from the stomach with colic and abdominal distension. Diarrhoea may occur.

Renal System. Scanty urination is dependent on a paralytic state of the bladder musculature.

Extremities. Twitching occurs in all muscles.

USES

This remedy has proved effective as adjunct therapy in grass tetany preventing brain damage when given in conjunction with conventional treatment. Hysteria in the dog will benefit in most cases. Post-distemper encephalitis and chorea may benefit and it should be remembered in this connection along with other remedies such as Belladonna.

Head-shaking in the horse may respond well. Brain conditions which call for its use are not generally accompanied by inflammation (unlike those conditions calling for Belladonna).

Hypericum Perforatum

St. John's Wort.   *N.O.* Hyperiaceae.   The Ø is prepared from the whole fresh plant.

The active principle is capable of causing sensitivity to light on some skin in the absence of melanin pigment. The main affinity of the plant is with the peripheral nervous system, causing hypersensitivity.

Skin.   Sweating occurs with eczematous conditions. Sloughing and necrosis may develop.

Alimentary System.   A scraping sound may be heard from the throat. Liver dysfunction develops along with jaundice.

Extremities.   Muscular jerking with a disposition to pain and sensitivity over the lumbar and sacral regions.

USES

This remedy is of prime importance in the treatment of lacerated wounds where nerve-endings are damaged. In spinal injuries, especially of the coccygeal area it products excellent results. The specific action on the nervous system has decided its use in the treatment of wounds likely to lead to tetanus and in this connection it is usually alternated with Ledum. Given early it helps prevent spread of the toxin along the nerve sheath. The pain of open wounds is quickly dispelled by this remedy and it should be used externally as a 1/10 lotion. If abscess formation develops after a wound Hypericum will be found useful in hastening resolution and draining the area. Conditions affecting the spine, e.g. disc trouble in the Dachshund breed, are generally greatly improved when this remedy is employed.

Iberis

Bitter Candytuft.   *N.O.* Cruciferae.   The Ø is prepared from seeds.
This plant produces a state of nervous excitement, and it also has a marked action on the heart.

Cardiac System.   The pulse is full and irregular, with an interrupted rhythm. Dilation of the heart leads to deficient output with consequent dropsy of dependent areas, seen as brisket swelling with oedema of the limbs in horses and cattle and ascites in the dog.

Alimentary System.   The circulatory interference leads to liver trouble with tenderness over the hepatic region. Stools tend to be whitish or clay-coloured.

Nervous System.   Vertigo of varying degrees of severity.

Respiratory System.   Pulmonary congestion arises as a result of deficient heart action. This leads to laboured respiration.

USES

This remedy should be kept in mind as one of the useful aids in treating heart conditions where deficient output leads to dropsical states. Old dogs will specially benefit, particularly those showing an accompanying excitability. Indicated in palpitation with distress on exertion.

Ignatia

St Ignatius Bean.   *N.O.* Loganiceae.   The Ø is prepared from trituration of seeds.
Hysteria and clonic spasms come within the sphere of action of this plant. There are few objective symptoms to be noticed which might make it a commonly used remedy in veterinary practice.

USES

It may have a place in dealing with certain post-partum conditions of bitches due to deprivation of pups and in the treatment of animals which have been separated from their companions. It is also a useful remedy in chorea of nervous origin and in muscular twitchings which may be associated with parasitism. This remedy also has an affinity with rectal conditions in general, e.g. prolapse.

Iodum

Iodine.   The Element.   The Ø is prepared from alcholic tincture.

A 1% tincture is the strength used in the preparation of homoeopathic remedies. In large doses – Iodism – sinuses and eyes are at first involved leading to conjunctivitis and bronchitis. Iodine has a special affinity with the thyroid gland.

Muscular System.   Weakness and atrophy of muscles may follow excess intake of iodine.

Eyes.   Dilated pupils and exophthalmous may occur. Oedema of the eyelids is accompanied by lachrymation.

Respiratory System.   The upper air passages are involved leading to cough and bronchitis which is aggravated by heat.

Alimentary System.   Salivation and inflammation of gums are common. The mouth and tongue may show aphthous ulcers. There is enlargement of liver with jaundice, and the abdomen becomes tympanitic. A characteristic diarrhoea sets in, viz. pale and frothy containing fat globules. Ravenous hunger is present.

Glandular System.   The lymph glands become hard. This applies also to the mammary gland which ultimately becomes shrivelled.

Renal System.   There is increased urination, the urine being dark and strong-smelling. It shows a luminous pellicle on standing.

Skin.   Dry and withered-looking.

USES

Conditions which show a characteristic oppositeness of symptoms, e.g. hunger or anorexia, tissue hyperplasia or atrophy may need this remedy. It may be useful in ovarian dysfunction where low potencies should be used. In skin conditions it is usually employed in combination with sulphur and in respiratory with Arsenicum Album. Affections of the thyroid gland call for its consideration. It is a useful gland remedy in general. A keynote to its use is a state of ravenous appetite with a corresponding loss of condition.

Ipecacuanha

N.O. Rubiaceae.   The Ø is prepared from trituration of dried root.

The dried root of this plant is the source of this remedy. Emetine, an alkaloid, is its principal constituent producing emesis and expectoration.

Eyes.   Lachrymation and general irritation lead to conjunctivitis.

Respiratory System.   Nasal bleeding of bright red blood. Spasmodic cough develops with difficult breathing, bronchitis and emphysema.

Alimentary System.   In the dog and cat retching and vomiting may lead to collapse. There may be almost continuous vomiting. In all species there is slimy diarrhoea and possibly dysentery.

Female Genital System.   Bleeding of bright red blood occurs from the uterus. In nurse animals the milk may contain blood giving it a pink colour.

USES

Because of its specific action on the stomach this remedy should be considered in any condition of the dog and cat producing constant vomition. It is also indicated in diarrhoea of young animals with a tendency to dysentery showing whole blood, e.g. as in coccidiosis of calves. It is a valuable anti-haemorrhagic remedy when the blood is bright red, especially uterine bleeding, post-partum. It has been used successfully in the treatment of cows showing blood-tinged milk. It could prove of value in suffocative breathing of old dogs. Some forms of coli-bacillosis in young calves may need it, especially those forms showing tenesmus with greenish stools. Symptoms of illness suggesting its use tend to come on quickly.

Iris Versicolor

Blue Flag.   *N.O.* Iridaceae.   The Ø is prepared from fresh root.

This plant produces an action on various glands, principally the salivary intestinal, pancreas and thyroid. It has a reputation also for aiding the secretion of bile.

Alimentary System.   Due to its action on the thyroid gland, swelling of the throat may occur. Vomiting of biliary material takes place in the dog and cat. There is usually lack of appetite, while colic and diarrhoea accompany tenderness over the liver region.

USES

The remedy may be indicated to control sluggish action of the liver, and may help counteract a tendency to jaundice. Its action on the pancreas suggests that it may be beneficial in some cases of diabetes. The general involvement of the alimentary canal may point to its use in such conditions as watery diarrhoea with colic and straining. It has a certain action on the skin and could be of use in eczema accompanying alimentary upsets. It has an action also on salivary glands and can be used to control some types of vomiting in dog and cat.

Jalapa

Exogonium Pursa. *N.O.* Convolvulaceae. The Ø is prepared from trituration of root.

A watery diarrhoea accompanied by colicky pains is the main symptom associated with this plant.

Alimentary System. The tongue is smooth, dry and glazed looking. Flatulence and diarrhoea occur, the latter being watery and muddy-looking.

USES

It should be remembered as a useful remedy in intestinal states showing the typical diarrhoea. It could be of service in colicky conditions associated with purging due to eating unsuitable food.

Juglans Cinerea

Butternut. *N.O.* Juglandaceae. The Ø is prepared from tincture of bark of root.

This plant produces a tendency to bile-stones and jaundice, together with eczematous skin conditions.

Alimentary System. Flatulence and distension commonly occur. The region over the liver is tender to the touch. Involvement of liver function leads to jaundice with gall-stone formation. Diarrhoea when it occurs is yellowish and pasty.

Back and Extremities. Pain is evident over the lumbar vertebrae while rigidity of neck muscles is a common feature.

Skin. The lower limbs and skin of the sacral region may show eczematous eruptions.

USES

A useful remedy in sluggish liver conditions showing jaundice with eczema. Its action on the skin may determine its use over competing liver remedies.

Juniperus

Juniper Berries.   *N.O.* from Coniferae.   The Ø is prepared from fresh ripe berries.

Juniper exerts its main action on the kidneys. It is especially adapted to older subjects.

Renal System.   The urine is scanty and blood-stained, and the animal has difficulty in passing it. The kidney substance becomes inflamed, an oedematous inflammation being established which leads to catarrhal discharges through the bladder and urethra. A common result is pyelitis.

USES

Both acute and chronic kidney conditions may call for its use. It has an action resembling to a lesser degree that of Cantharis, but the symptoms are much more violent in the latter. Also skin symptoms are invariably absent in conditions suggesting Juniperus. Urine containing pus may suggest pyelitis which is occasionally met with in cattle and here we should consider high potencies ranging from 200c to 10m. Cystitis in dogs and cats is a fairly common condition which may need this remedy in preference to others.

Kali Arsenicum

Fowler's Solution.   The Ø is prepared from arsenious acid and potassium carbonate solution.

The main action of this salt which concerns us in the veterinary sphere is exerted on the skin with a tendency to malignancy of the internal organs.

Skin.   A dry scaly eczema is set up with severe itching. This condition is often long-standing. Slow-healing ulcers appear with fissures in the region of the elbows and hock.

USES

This is a very useful remedy in chronic eczematous conditions. It may give better results than Arsenicum Album when the latter is seemingly indicated in skin disorders. It has been used successfully in sweet-itch in the horse and is often combined or alternated with Sulphur Iodatum. It could have a place in the treatment of possible early malignancy in the older animal and should be considered if treatment is requested.

Kali Bichromicum

Potassium Dichromate.   The Ø is prepared from solution in water (distilled).

This potassium salt acts on the mucous membranes of the stomach, intestines and respiratory tract with lesser involvement of other organs. Feverish states are absent. Also characteristic is anaemia and lassitude. The action on the mucous membranes produces a catarrh of a tough, stringy nature with a yellowish colour.

Eyes.   Catarrhal discharges with oedema of eyelids. Ulceration of cornea.

Ears.   Thick discharge with unpleasant smell.

Respiratory System.   Catarrhal inflammation of sinuses leading to discharges which are thick and stringy. Profuse yellow expectoration.

Alimentary System.   Inflammation of stomach producing

retching and vomiting in the dog and cat. This is often relieved by eating. Stools are glutinous and blood-stained.

Renal System. Nephritis and pyelitis. Urine may contain mucus, pus and blood.

Female Genital System. Yellowish catarrhal discharge from uterus.

Skin. Papular eruptions with ulcer formation.

USES

Tough, yellow, stringy discharges are strong indications for the use of this remedy. This applies to all mucous surfaces and it should be remembered in such conditions as broncho-pneumonia, purulent sinusitis and pyelitis, where the character of the discharges suggest it, a strong guiding symptom being the yellowish colour. It may have a use in some forms of pyometra. Ulcerative conditions of the skin come within its sphere of action, the ulcers being round with clean-cut edges. It has been used successfully in lymphangitis, cellulitis and grease in the horse. Corneal ulcer may benefit and in this connection it may also be used in the form of a lotion, diluted 1/200.

Kali Carbonicum

Potassium Carbonate. The Ø is prepared from solution in distilled water.

This salt is found in all plants and in the soil, the colloid material of cells containing the element. It produces a generalised weakness which is common to other potassium salts. Feverish states are absent.

Eyes. Oedematous, puffy swellings appear on upper eyelids.

Alimentary System. Swelling of tonsils takes place along with firmness of parotid glands. Liver function is interfered with and there may be jaundice. In the dog and cat vomition occurs, while inflammation of the stomach occurs in all species. Abdominal tympany occurs and stools are passed with difficulty.

Skin. There is excessive dryness with falling of hair in older subjects.

Renal System. Urination is difficult and the urine generally contains salts, especially urates.

Muscular System. Marked weakness appears in which the legs suddenly give way. Oedematous, doughy swellings appear at different places.

Cardiac System. A rapid weak pulse accompanies palpitation.

USES

This is mainly a remedy for the older dog and cat, especially in weakened states. It is useful after parturition or illness as a constitutional remedy, helping as it does to restore strength. It could be of use in animals showing sluggish liver function and may also benefit older dogs suffering from chronic kidney conditions. A main guiding symptom is the appearance of baggy swellings on the upper eyelids.

Kali Chloricum

Potassium Chlorate. The Ø is prepared from solution in distilled water.

The urinary organs are chiefly affected by this salt.

Alimentary System. Redness of the mouth with ulceration accompanies profuse salivation. In the dog and cat vomiting takes place. The mucous membrane of the large intestine becomes inflamed producing a diarrhoea of a greenish colour, containing mucus.

Renal System. Inflammation of the kidney substance takes place producing urine which is blood-stained and contains albumen. The phosphate content of the urine is high.

Skin. Uncovered areas appear yellowish, and papular eruptions occur on various sites.

USES

This is one of many remedies which should be thought of when dealing with the chronic and acute kidney complaints of dogs. The urine should be tested for high phosphate concentration which may help to decide its use over other remedies. There may also be abdominal symptoms present in these cases such as greenish slimy diarrhoea. Useful in controlling mouth ulcerations if these arise in conjunction with other symptoms.

Kali Hydriodicum

Potassium Iodide. The Ø is prepared from solution in distilled water.

This important drug produces an acrid, watery discharge from the eyes and also acts on fibrous and connective tissue. Glandular swellings appear with a tendency to purpura.

Eyes. Lachrymation first appears which leads on to inflammation of the cornea with possible ulceration and conjunctivitis.

Respiratory System. A thin, watery nasal discharge develops into a greenish catarrh. Dropsical conditions occur in various areas such as larynx, pleura and lungs, leading to difficulty in breathing.

Female Genital System. A sub-acute inflammation of the uterus takes place producing a whitish discharge.

Extremities. Stiffness of joints is associated with pain which causes the animal to cry out suddenly.

Skin. The superficial lymph glands become enlarged and indurated. Nodules occur on the skin and there may be oedematous swellings.

USES

This is a widely used remedy in various conditions showing the typical eye and respiratory conditions, e.g. pneumonia with effusion accompanied by coryza. It is beneficial in fog-fever in cattle and in New Forest Disease, where if given early it will arrest the progress of the disease and prevent damage to eye structures. It is one of the main remedies to be considered in actinobacillosis of cattle, especially when the sub-maxillary glands are involved, although it will also produce good results when the tongue alone is diseased. Thyroid swelling in the dog may also benefit.

Kali Muriaticum

Potassium Chloride. The Ø is prepared from the solution in distilled water.

Glandular swellings occur under the influence of this drug, with, in addition, expectoration of thick phlegm.

Respiratory System. Spasmodic cough occurs with expectoration of mucus.

Alimentary System. White ulcers appear in the mouth which develops a thick coating of the tongue. Tonsils become inflamed with fibrinous deposits. In the dog and cat mucous vomiting occurs. Dysentery is common with slimy mucus.

Skin. Bran-like flakes occur on the skin, with occasionally a vesicular eczema.

USES

Glandular swellings in general and catarrhal conditions come within the sphere of action of this remedy, and it could prove of value in dysenteric and pulmonary inflammations. It may be useful in the early stages of canine hepatitis where swelling of sub-maxillary and parotid glands take place. Might prove useful in early Hodgkin's disease and also in affection of ears.

Kali Nitricum

Potassium Nitrate. This is a valuable remedy in conditions affecting

chest and heart. There is also a marked action on the alimentary and
urinary systems.

Alimentary System.   Red tongue, showing papular eruptions.
Dysenteric stools with shreds of mucous membrane.

Respiratory System.   Bronchitis leads to cough with expectoration of blood.

Cardiac System.   The pulse is weak and thready.

Renal System.   Various types of nephritis may be seen.

USES

This is a useful remedy in bronchitis with dry cough and conditions
which produce oedematous swellings. Also in gastro-intestinal affections and nephritis. Diabetes insipidus may benefit.

Kali Phosphoricum

Potassium Phosphate.   The Ø is prepared from solution in distilled
water.

This salt produces prostration and disturbances of the sympathetic
nervous system.

Respiratory System.   Nasal discharge dependent on disease of
the nasal mucosa. There is shortness of breath and cough with yellow
expectoration.

Eyes.   Weakness of eye muscles leads to drooping of eyelids.

Alimentary System.   Dryness of mouth accompanies a coated
tongue and bleeding of gums. There may be a putrid diarrhoea with
possibly dysentery.

Renal System.   Yellowish urine with urethral bleeding.

Extremities.   Weakness of back and lower limbs.

USES

This remedy has a place in the treatment of suspected early tumour
formation. It helps restore strength in debilitated conditions and is more
adapted to the young subject in generalised weakness.

Kali Sulphuricum

Potassium Sulphate.   The Ø is prepared from solution in distilled
water.

The later stages of inflammation are influenced by this remedy. It
produces mucous and serous discharges, sometimes profuse and yellow.

Respiratory System.   Posterior inflammation of nasal passages, rattling of mucus in the chest, yellow expectoration with cough which becomes worse in the evening.

Alimentary System. Thirst is prominent. In the dog and cat vomiting occurs. Slimy diarrhoea, yellowish in colour.

Skin. Papular eruptions occur. There may be desquamation of surface scales.

USES

This remedy has a place in the treatment of broncho-pneumonia. Certain types of ringworm may benefit and also eczema where the skin shows desquamation. It could be of value in mucosal disease of calves when there is respiratory involvement as well as bowel symptoms.

Kalmia Latifolia

Mountain Laurel. *N.O.* Ericaceae. The Ø is prepared from fresh leaves.

This plant has a prominent action on the heart. Large doses of the active principle reduces the general action considerably.

Alimentary System. Vomiting occurs in the dog and cat, while bilious attacks frequently take place.

Renal System. Nephritis takes place with albuminuria. Urination is frequent. The lumbar region is sensitive to pressure.

Cardiac System. The pulse is weak. Palpitation is accompanied by fibrillation.

Respiratory System. Because of the weak heart action there is a general shortness of breath.

Extremities. Joints of the legs become stiff. Muscular tenseness and hardness may appear.

USES

This remedy may be of use in heart conditions of old dogs, especially those showing a slowness of action. Joint conditions of the older dog may also benefit. Dropsical states, e.g. ascites, should benefit and it may benefit nephritic cases indirectly.

Kreosotum

Beechwood Kreosote. The Ø is prepared from solution in rectified spirit.

This substance produces haemorrhages from small wounds with burning discharges and ulcerations. It also causes rapid decomposition of fluids.

Eyes.   Inflammation of eyelids, sometimes chronic. The eyelids become red and itching may be severe.

Ears.   The external ear becomes hot accompanied by eruptions and pimply ulceration.

Extremities.   The neck becomes stiff.

Skin.   There is a tendency to gangrene. Ulceration and bleeding of small wounds takes place. There may be a vesicular-type eruption.

Renal System.   Frequency of urination. Copious pale urine which may change to dark with a turbid appearance.

Alimentary System.   Rapid decay of teeth with spongy bleeding gums. There may be bleeding from the stomach and diarrhoea of black putrid material.

Female Genital System.   Bleeding of dark blood from uterus.

USES

This is a useful remedy in threatened gangrenous conditions arising from putrid or septic states, e.g. haemorrhagic pneumonia. Ulcerations and eruptions of the skin come within its sphere of action. It could be of value in putrid conditions of the mouth with haemorrhagic decay of teeth. It has been used with success in uraemic conditions of dogs showing the characteristic putrid discharges and smoky urine. In young animals a clue to its use would be early decay of teeth after eruption.

Lac Caninum

Milk of the Bitch.   The Ø is prepared from whole milk.

This substance increases the flow of milk in material doses and also produces sore throat and rheumatic-like pains.

Respiratory System. Purulent nasal discharges with watery coryza at times.

Alimentary System. Salivation is common and the tongue is coated white with red edges. The throat becomes inflamed resulting in difficulty in swallowing. A membranous deposit shows on the back of the tongue. This deposit may appear first on one side and then on the other.

Female Genital System. The mammary glands become enlarged and painful, and the milk flow is increased.

USES

Its action on the mammary glands determines its main use in veterinary practice. It should always be considered in false pregnancy to control the secretion of milk. It will aid the return of the udder to normal after weaning or removal of unwanted pups. The throat symptoms suggest that it may be of use in pharyngitis or tonsillitis and in this connection it could be useful in calf diptheria.

Lachesis

Bushmaster venom.   The Ø is prepared from dilution in alcohol.

This venom produces decomposition of blood, rendering it more fluid. There is a strong tendency to haemorrhages and septic states with profound prostration.

Respiratory System. Bleeding from the nose with coryza in less severe cases.

Alimentary System. The tongue becomes swollen and the gums bleed. This swelling extends to the throat which shows sepsis, a purple livid colour developing. The abdomen is swollen and sensitive, and bleeding occurs from the lower intestine.

Female Genital System. The mammary glands are inflamed and purplish. Fluid black blood comes from the uterus.

Cardiac System. The pulse is weak. Cyanosis develops producing a dusky appearance on the tongue and visible mucous membranes.

Skin. This assumes a bluish appearance. Boils and carbuncles develop with purplish edges. Wounds become septic with necrotic black edges. Inflammation extends to deeper tissues producing a cellulitis with swollen lymphatics.

USES

This is a useful remedy in adder bites, helping to prevent septic involvement and reducing swelling. It is particularly valuable if the throat region develops inflammatory lesions causing swelling. In this connection the left side of the throat including the parotid gland is more severely affected than the right where haemorrhagic conditions arise. The blood is dark and does not clot readily. The remedy may be called for in puerperal sepsis showing typical blood-stained discharges and purplish or bluish discolouration of abdominal skin. In these we would expect the mammary glands to show swelling and discolouration with again the left side being more heavily involved.

Lathyrus

Chick Pea. *N.O.* Leguminosae. The Ø is prepared from the flower or pods.

This drug affects the anterior columns of the spinal cord, producing paralysis of the lower extremities. Nerve power generally is weakened and this may involve various areas.

Renal System. Urination becomes frequent but there may be weakness in expulsion because of partial paralysis of nerves supplying the bladder musculature.

Extremities. Rigidity of muscles develops producing a weak, tottery gait. Paralysis of nerves in turn produces wasting of various groups of muscles, especially the gluteal and those of the lower limbs. Initially the legs may show swelling.

Respiratory System. If nerves controlling respiration become involved distress in breathing becomes evident, causing the animal to exhibit symptoms of air hunger.

Alimentary System. Inability to swallow properly may follow weakness of muscles of the throat. Consequently there may be drooling of saliva. Constipation usually develops because of the loss of expulsive power and involvement of nerve-endings in the gut.

USES

This remedy may be useful in the treatment of some forms of post-distemper paralysis, and rivals Conium in this respect. In equine practice it could be worth trying in the generally considered hopeless disease – grass sickness. The weakness and heaviness of post-influenzal conditions may benefit and in this disease it compares favourably with Gelsemium when symptoms of local paralysis develop. It may also be of use in the condition known as roaring due to weakness or paralysis of certain muscles of the larynx and this approach should be thoroughly explored before surgery is contemplated. Urinary incontinence due to local weakness of bladder musculature should benefit.

Laurocerasus

Cherry Laurel.　*N.O.* Rosaceae.　The Ø is prepared from fresh young leaves.

This shrub produces heart symptoms associated with a tickling cough. Cyanosis usually develops and there is a generally cold feeling to the touch.

Respiratory System. Difficulty in breathing. Exercise produces distress, a dry cough developing.

Cardiac System. The valves are chiefly affected, mitral regurgitation being the chief pathological condition. This produces a cyanotic condition with a small feeble pulse.

Extremities. Stiffness and pain develop in the lower limbs. Superficial veins become distended.

USES

Valvular disease in the older dog may benefit from this remedy. The animal is usually presented with signs of cyanosis and a typical dry cough with respiratory distress.

Ledum Palustre

Marsh Tea.　*N.O.* Ericaceae.　The Ø is prepared from the whole fresh plant.

The active principle of this plant produces tetanus-like symptoms with twitching of muscles along with rheumatic pains.

Respiratory System. Nose bleeding occurs along with blood-stained cough. Breathing becomes difficult on account of bronchitis and emphysema. Pressure over the chest wall causes resentment. A spasmodic action occurs in the muscles of respiration with double-action inspiration.

Skin.   There is a tendency to bluish discolouration after injuries.
Eczema may occur with possibly small cutaneous haemorrhages.
Extremities.   These become swollen and the feet feel hot. There
is tenderness and stiffness over the shoulder area.

USES

This is one of the main remedies for consideration in cases of punctured
wounds. Given along with Hypericum it helps prevent tetanus. It is especially indicated when the surrounding parts are bluish and cold. Its action
on the respiratory system suggests its use in emphysema. It is also a useful eye remedy in such conditions as corneal ulcers and conjunctivitis.

Lemna Minor

Duckweed.   *N.O.* Lemnaceae.   The Ø is prepared from whole fresh
plants.
     This is a remedy for catarrhal conditions affecting mainly the nasal
passages.
Respiratory System.   A muco-purulent nasal discharge develops. It helps reduce nasal obstruction.
Alimentary System.   Dryness of mouth and throat. The intestinal mucous membrane may develop catarrhal inflammation leading to
diarrhoea accompanied by flatulence.

USES

Rhinitis should benefit from the use of this remedy and it could be of service in many conditions where catarrhal inflammation is a prominent
symptom. There is usually a history of muco-purulent sometimes blood-
stained discharge which could be due to polypus formation.

Leptandra

Culver's Root.   *N.O.* Scrophulariaceae.   The Ø is prepared from dried
root.
     This is a prominent liver remedy producing many of the symptoms
of disturbances of the portal system.
Alimentary System.   Clay-coloured diarrhoea with signs of
jaundice followed by profuse black stools. There is a tendency to rectal
prolapse. Jaundice produces a yellowish discolouration of tongue. The
animal resents pressure over the liver area.

USES

This is a useful remedy in affections of the liver where jaundice is

evident and blackish stools are present. It could have a use in canine
hepatitis and jaundice.

Liatris Spicata

Colic Root.   *N.O.* Compositae.   The Ø is prepared from the powdered fresh root.
This is mainly a digestive and urinary remedy. It promotes digestion and has a beneficial action on the liver, stimulating the portal circulation and thereby reducing any abdominal fluid present.

USES
Should be remembered as a digestive stimulant, and could be useful in
various colicky conditions. It is also one of the remedies useful in diarrhoea accompanied by cramp-like behaviour.

Lilium Tigrinum

Tiger Lily.   *N.O.* Liliaceae.   The Ø is prepared from fresh leaves and
flowers.
The action is mainly on the pelvic organs producing conditions
which arise from uterine or ovarian disturbance.
Eyes.   Lachrymation first occurs. It helps restore power to weakened ciliary muscles.
Alimentary System.   There is thirst for small amounts of water.
A distended abdomen accompanies flatulence. Dysentery may occur.
Renal System.   The urine is scanty and there is frequent passage.
Cardiac System.   The heart rate is increased and a rapid irregular pulse arises.
Female Genital System.   Congestion and blood-stained discharge from the uterus. There may be prolapse. Inflammation of
ovaries.

USES
It is mainly of use in uterine and ovarian conditions. Pyometra and the
various forms of infertility in cattle may respond when other remedies
fail, especially those involving ovarian function.

Lithium Carbonicum

Lithium Carbonate.   The Ø is prepared from trituration of dried salt.

This salt produces a chronic rheumatic-like state with a uric acid diathesis. It also has an action on the heart.

Eyes. The eyelids become dry due to diminished lachrymal secretion. There is aversion to light.

Alimentary System. Symptoms of gastric and abdominal discomfort such as vomition in the dog and tympany in general are relieved by eating.

Renal System. There is difficulty in passing urine, which contains mucus and a red sandy deposit. Cystitis develops, the urine being dark.

Extremities. Rheumatic-like stiffness and affections of joints, especially carpal and metacarpal in the fore-limbs and the hock and metatarsals in the hind.

Skin. An erythematous rash may develop into an eczema with the production of loose flakes.

USES

It should be remembered as a useful addition to the other remedies which are of value in cystitis and nephritis with uric acid formation. Rheumatism of small joints, especially in the older dog may benefit. Its specific action on the skin should be noted.

Lobelia Inflata

Indian Tobacco.   *N.O.* Lobeliaceae.   The Ø is prepared from dried leaves.

The active principle of this plant acts as a vaso-motor stimulant impeding respiration and producing symptoms of nausea with vomiting and relaxation of muscles.

Alimentary System. Profuse salivation accompanies abdominal flatulence. In the dog and cat vomiting readily takes place. After eating respiration becomes difficult, probably due to gastric tympany.

Respiratory System. Breathing is generally difficult. Exertion produces coughing and in the older animal emphysema develops.

Renal System. The urine becomes dark with a heavy red sediment.

USES

Languor with muscular relaxation is a main indication for the use of this remedy. It should prove useful when given as a convalescent aid after influenza in the horse. Specific conditions which may benefit include emphysema and gastric upsets in the dog and cat. It might prove useful in incontinent states of the older dog.

Lycopodium

Club Moss. *N.O.* Lycopodiaceae. The Ø is prepared from spores or from the whole plant.

The spores of this plant contain its active principle which acts chiefly on the renal and digestive systems. There is a tendency to the production of renal calculi. The respiratory system is also markedly affected.

Eyes. Redness of eyelids accompanies a tendency to corneal ulceration.

Ears. Eczema occurs behind the ear. The ears themselves may discharge thick yellow material.

Respiratory System. Profuse watery nasal secretion. The nostrils show a typical fan-like motion which is independent of respiration. Coughing and difficult breathing are common features while pneumonia frequently develops.

Alimentary System. Salivation occurs with blisters on the tongue. The throat becomes inflamed and tonsillar ulceration develops. There is a general lack of gastric function and very little food is seen to satisfy the animal. The abdomen becomes bloated with tenderness over the liver region. The liver itself may become inflamed and lead to ascites and hard stools.

Renal System. The urine may become retained due to sluggish action on the part of the urinary tract. A heavy red sediment occurs which is the precursor of kidney and bladder calculi.

Cardiac System. Palpitation occurs with signs of arterial tension such as throbbing of superficial vessels, e.g. the carotid arteries.

Extremities. The tendency to calculi formation may lead to the deposition of uric acid crystals in the joints.

Skin. There is a tendency to ulceration and fissured eruptions. A chronic eczema may develop.

USES

This is a useful remedy in various digestive and respiratory conditions. Acetonaemia in cattle is greatly helped. Hepatitis and abdominal disorders with sand in the urine may be secondary to liver disturbance. Pregnancy toxaemia in the ewe may respond to its use if treatment is started early enough. Its action on the skin suggest its use in dried-up or withered looking conditions and it has been used with success in alopecia. Chronic colicky conditions in the horse accompanied by hard slimy dung may respond favourably and it could be indicated also in depraved appetite in this species.

Lycopus Virginicus

Bugle Weed.   *N.O.* Labiatae.   The Ø is prepared from fresh whole plant.

The active principle of this plant reduces blood-pressure and causes passive haemorrhages.

Eyes.   There is a tendency to protrusion of the eyeball.

Cardiac Region.   The pulse becomes weak and irregular. The heart action is increased and is accompanied by difficult breathing and signs of cyanosis.

Respiratory System.   The breathing assumes a wheezy character and may produce a blood-tinged cough.

Renal System.   There is an abundance of pale urine with a tendency to diabetes insipidus.

USES

This is a valuable remedy in certain forms of heart disease, especially when associated with asthmatic symptoms and blood-stained expectoration. It will be seen therefore to play a useful part in canine practice for the treatment of the older dog, more especially as these cases are frequently associated with degenerative kidney disease.

Magnesia Carbonica

Magnesium Carbonate.   The Ø is prepared from trituration of dried salt.

This salt produces catarrhal inflammation of the gastro-intestinal tract with a tendency to sensitivity of the nervous system.

Ears.   The animal may show signs of diminished hearing.

Alimentary System.   A dry mouth is accompanied by vesicular eruptions. Any saliva which is produced may be blood-stained. Diarrhoea develops which is green and watery, containing blood-stained mucus.

Respiratory System.   Breathing is laboured with expectoration containing blood.

USES

Certain forms of coli-bacillosis of young animals may need this remedy when the typical stools are present. The action on the mouth accompanying changes in the intestinal canal suggests its use in mucosal disease of calves. It this respect respiratory involvement may also occur suggesting a further reason for its use. Nervous dogs may benefit from it use especially gun-shy animals and those sensitive to noise.

Magnesia Muriatica

Magnesium Chloride.   The Ø is prepared from solution in distilled water.

This salt produces marked inactivity of the bowels and digestive upsets.

Respiratory System.   Nasal discharge of watery material together with ulceration of nostrils.

Alimentary System.   Blisters develop around the mouth. Gums become swollen and bleed easily. The tongue is usually discoloured with a yellow coating. There is an inability to digest milk. Enlargement of the liver is accompanied by abdominal bloating and pressure on the abdomen may produce urination. Young animals show a strong disposition to firmness of stools.

Renal System.   There is difficulty in urinating, great pressure being needed to empty the bladder.

USES

Mainly of use in liver and abdominal affections leading to inactivity of the bowels especially in chronic affections.

Magnesia Phosphorica

Magnesium Phosphate.   The Ø is prepared from solution in distilled water.

This drug acts on muscles producing a cramping effect with spasm.

Head.   Vertigo with a tendency to fall forward.

Eyes.   Twitching of eyelids which become heavy and drooping. Lachrymation develops.

Alimentary System.   The throat and associated glands become swollen and stiff. Colicky pains develop causing the animal to paw or kick at the abdomen.

Extremities.   Involuntary twitching of the legs occurs. There is a general tendency to nervous chorea-like movement.

USES

This is a valuable remedy to be remembered in treating cases of hypo-magnesaemia in cattle and sheep, where its prompt use will help prevent brain damage. It may be given along with standard injections in this connection. It is also one of the remedies which may be needed in colic and abdominal tympany.

Magnesia Sulphurica

Magnesium Sulphate.   The Ø is prepared from trituration of salt.

This salt – commonly known as Epsom's Salts – produces a marked action on the intestinal canal, the urinary system and the skin.

Alimentary System.   A watery diarrhoea develops mainly due to the physical action of the drug on the bowel wall.

Renal System.   The urine becomes bright yellow showing a high turbidity. Output is increased and there develops a red sediment.

Female Genital System.   Vaginal discharges develop which are profuse, thick and of a catarrhal nature.

Skin.   A papular rash occurs with wart formation.

USES

Certain forms of nephritis may benefit especially those associated with turbid reddish sediment in the urine. In canine practice it could have a use in the treatment of diabetes.

Manganum Aceticum

Manganese Acetate. The Ø is prepared from solution in distilled water.

This salt causes anaemia with destruction of red blood-corpuscles.

Respiratory System. Laryngitis develops with difficult expectoration which becomes worse towards evening. Cough may be bloodstained.

Extremities. Muscular twitching with stiffness. Joints become swollen.

Skin. There is a tendency to an itching suppurative state around joints.

Alimentary System. Ulceration of the tongue takes place with the appearance of warty growths. Liver troubles are common in the form of chronic hepatitis leading to flatulence and jaundice.

USES

This is a useful remedy in degenerative anaemic states with a tendency to liver involvement. Cellulitis may respond to its use, especially when there is an accompanying suppuration. In cattle practice it has a special place in the treatment of some forms of infertility which are associated with trace element deficiency, manganese frequently being implicated. Periostitis should also benefit and the action on the liver suggests its possible use in hepatitis. It may be indicated in some types of dry itching of the skin.

Melilotus

Sweet Clover. *N.O.* Leguminoseae. The Ø is prepared from whole fresh plant.

The active principle of this plant is capable of producing congestions leading to haemorrhage. The clotting power of the blood is interfered with.

Respiratory System. Nasal bleeding may be profuse. Haemorrhage from the lungs is also commonplace, the blood being bright red.

Extremities. The carpal joints show evidence of pain, possibly because of bleeding into the joint. The skin becomes cold.

USES

This is a very useful remedy in haemorrhagic states especially after mechanical trauma, e.g. haematoma. Subcutaneous bleeding of unknown origin may find a useful aid in this remedy.

Mercurius Corrosivus

Corrosive Sublimate.　The Ø is prepared from trituration of the salt.

Mercuric chloride produces tenesmus of the lower bowel and also has a destructive action on kidney tissue.

Eyes.　Acrid water discharges. Inflammation of the iris without suppuration. Eyelids become oedematous, red and excoriated.

Respiratory System.　Excessive mucous discharges from nose. Coughing with bleeding from lungs.

Ears.　Inflammation mainly of outer ear with purulent discharge.

Alimentary System.　The tongue is swollen and inflamed. Salivation is copious. Throat is red and swollen. In the dog and cat there may be vomiting of greenish bile. Dysentery is a constant feature and is accompanied by pronounced tenesmus which is not relieved by passing stool.

Renal System.　Urine is usually suppressed. Chronic nephritis is common, with production of blood-stained albuminous urine.

Male Genital System.　Swelling of penis and testicles.

USES

This again is a very frequently indicated remedy, especially is small animal practice, e.g. in chronic nephritis and dysenteric states. Cat 'flu has responded well to its use. Although it has no specific action on the skin it has been found in practice to be of great benefit in wet eczema when this occurs as part of a constitutional breakdown and in this connection chronic otitis externa is also greatly benefited.

Mercurius Cyanatus

Cyanide of Mercury.　The Ø is prepared from solution in distilled water.

This salt produces an action similar to that of bacterial toxins. Haemorrhagic tendency and prostration are common features.

Alimentary System.　Ulceration of the mucous membranes of mouth and throat are pronounced features. The tongue is pale and salivary glands are swollen and tender. A greyish membrane surrounds ulcers which form on the throat and in the mouth. The pharyngeal region is one of the main areas affected, redness of the mucous membranes preceding necrosis in the later stages. Dysentery may be present with pronounced straining. The stools are dark and have a gangrenous odour. In the dog and cat vomiting of blood-stained bile occurs. The abdominal area is tender to the touch.

Renal System. The urine is scanty, albuminous and dark golden in colour.

USES

The value of this remedy lies in its relation to certain types of septic inflammations, especially pronounced in the mouth and throat. It may prove useful in some forms of nephritis with suppression and threatened uraemia. More specifically calf-diphtheria is one condition where it has proved of use.

Mercurius Dulcis

Calomel. The Ø is prepared from trituration of the salt.

The mercurous chloride of mercury produces a marked effect on the middle ear, causing catarrhal inflammation. The liver is also affected.

Ears. Inflammation of middle and external ear producing catarrhal discharge.

Alimentary System. Salivation is prominent. The tongue becomes black and ulcerated. In the dog and cat bilious vomiting occurs. Stools are scanty with blood-stained mucus. Hepatitis and accompanying jaundice result from the action on the liver. This may produce a feverish, bilious condition.

Skin. Dark-coloured eruptions occur which show a tendency to ulceration.

USES

This remedy has some value in liver cirrhosis with attendant dropsy, and in conditions showing bilious remissions. Ear canker in dogs and cats may call for its use and it has been used successfully in mucous colitis.

Mercurius Iodatus Flavus

Yellow Iodide of Mercury. The Ø is prepared from trituration of the salt.

Mercurius iodide produces a tendency to glandular induration with attendant coating of the tongue.

Alimentary System. The tongue becomes coated, assuming a yellowish discolouration. Submaxillary and parotid glands may become swollen, especially on the right side. Tonsillitis is frequently present.

USES

Various swellings of glandular tissue come within the sphere of this remedy, e.g. parotitis and lymphadenitis generally. It could be useful in actinobacillosis of throat glands and in mild mammary tumour in the bitch.

Mercurius Iodatus Ruber

Red Iodide of Mercury.   The Ø is prepared from·trituration of the salt.

Mercuric iodide also shows a tendency to glandular involvement, but these usually begin on the left side.

Alimentary System.   The throat is dark red and swollen. Stiffness of neck muscles sets in because of swelling of left sub-maxillary and parotid glands.

Respiratory System.   Nasal discharge of mucoid material.

Skin.   Hard papules may develop with a tendency to ulcerate producing a local sepsis.

USES

This is a useful remedy to remember in chronic suppurating states with throat involvement. It could prove of value in calf-diptheria and in the early stages of canine hepatitis.

Mercurius Solubilis

Mercury.   The Ø is prepared from trituration of element.

The metal mercury affects most organs of the body producing cellular degeneration with consequent anaemic states.

Eyes.   Swollen eyelids accompany acrid purulent discharges. Generalised conjunctivitis.

Ears.   Inflammation of inner and outer ear. Evil smelling purulent discharges.

Respiratory System.   Ulceration of nasal septum and nostrils leading to purulent coryza. Muco-purulent expectoration with coughing.

Alimentary System.   Salivation is profuse and frequently blood-stained. Gums become spongy and teeth loosen, with a tendency to abscess formation. Thirst is present despite the wet mouth. The liver becomes enlarged with jaundice and flatulence frequent sequelae. Diarrhoea is slimy and blood-stained.

Renal System.   Chronic Bright's Disease produces dark albuminous urine.

Skin.   There is a tendency to ulceration. Eruptions range from pimply to vesicular.

Extremities.   Twitching of muscles. Tremulous gait. Dropsical swellings.

USES

This is an indispensible remedy and may be needed for almost any condition met with in canine practice, ranging from ear canker to dysentery, hepatis and nephritis. Conditions calling for its use are generally worse during the hours from sunset to sunrise. A strong guiding symptom for its consideration is abundance of slimy saliva.

Mezereum

Spurge Olive.   *N.O.* Thymelaceae.   The Ø is prepared from fresh bark.

The active principle of this plant produces symptoms of skin involvement together with intestinal affections.

Skin.   Eczema occurs with severe itching. Vesicles arise which progress to ulcer formation with a surrounding red area. When scabs form they tend to become under-run with pus.

Uro-Genital System.   Nephritis occurs with the appearance of blood in the urine. In the male testicular swelling may arise.

Alimentary System.   In the dog and cat vomiting occurs. Generalised gastro-enteritis. Flatulence and colicky pains develop.

USES

Principally of use in eczematous conditions, especially of the face and head. The lesions are crusty with sticky purulent discharges underneath.

Millefolium

Yarrow.   *N.O.* Compositae.   The Ø is prepared from whole fresh plant.

Haemorrhages occur from various parts from the action of this plant, the blood being bright red.

Respiratory System.   Nasal bleeding. Cough with bleeding from lungs.

Alimentary System.   Haemorrhages of bright red blood from the bowels.

Renal System.   Bleeding may occur from any portion of the urinary tract.

Female Genital System.   Post-partum, the uterus may be the seat of vascular weakness producing flow of bright red blood.

USES

Because of its ability to produce extensive haemorrhages it could be of value in the treatment of warfarin poisoning. It should not be used in too high a potency.

Morphinum

The Alkaloid Morphine.   The Ø is prepared from solution in distilled water.

This alkaloid produces a marked hypnotic state with less convulsant states than its source – opium.

Head.   Vertigo occurs with the least movement. There is a tendency to draw the head backwards.

Eyes.   Drooping of eyelids. Pupils assume a fixed look. Cornea appears reddish due to enlargement and engorgement of eye vessels.

Alimentary System.   In the dog and cat there is vomiting of bilious material. The abdomen becomes distended.

Renal System.   Difficulty in urination. Tendency to suppression with threatened uraemia.

Respiratory System.   Breathing becomes difficult with a dry cough.

Skin.   Urticaria occurs with herpetic eruptions.

USES

It could prove of value in comatose states, especially if accompanied by skin lesions. The eye symptoms could be the main attendant guide.

Murex

Purple Fish.   The Ø is prepared from dried juice.

The substance used is the dried secretion of the purple gland of one of the murex species. It exerts its action mainly on the female genital system, producing irregularities of the oestrus cycle.

Renal System.   There is a tendency to frequent urination.

Female Genital System.   There may be partial prolapse of the uterus Uterine discharge of blood-stained material accompanies a chronic inflammatory state.

USES

This remedy has been used mainly in cattle practice where it has proved useful in regulating the oestrus cycle. It has been employed both in anoestrus and for stimulating ovulation and for cystic ovaries.

Muriatic Acid

Hydrochloric Acid. The Ø is prepared from solution in distilled water.

This acid produces a blood condition analogous to that produced by septic feverish conditions of a chronic nature. There is a tendency to the formation of ulcers.

Respiratory System. Nasal bleeding.

Alimentary System. Ulceration of lips, with swollen gums and neck glands. The throat becomes dark red and oedematous. There may be evacuation of bowels associated with passing of urine.

Cardiac Region. The pulse is small and rapid.

Extremities. Movements are laboured with a weak gait.

Skin. Eruptions vary from papular to vesicular. The lower parts of the front legs are frequently the seat of foul-smelling ulcers.

USES

It should be considered in low-grade inflammatory conditions with a tendency to haemorrhage. Eczema of the limbs calls for its consideration and in this connection it could be of use in the treatment of ulcerative lymphangitis and allied conditions. Epithelioma and rodent ulcers (e.g. in the cat) may improve under its long-term use. Mouth ulcers in general along with apthal sordes on teeth.

Mygale Lasidora

Black Cuban Spider. The Ø is prepared from tincture of spider in alcohol.

The poison of this spider produces chorea-like symptoms in which weakness and palpitation predominate.

Head. Twitching of facial muscles develops. The mouth and eyes open in alternation, and there is difficulty in protrusion of the tongue.

Alimentary System. Thirst is excessive but aversion to food is usual.

Male Genital System.   Signs of increased sexual desire are common.

Extremities.   The animal walks unsteadily, with twitching of limbs. The entire body is restless, the patient moving about continually. Lymphatic vessels may become enlarged and show as red streaks. Movements are generally convulsive in character.

USES

Nervous conditions in general may find a use in this remedy, especially post-distemper chorea. Hypomagnesaemia in cattle and sheep may benefit in mild cases.

Myrica

Bayberry.   *N.O.* Myricaceae.   The Ø is prepared from fresh bark of root.

The active principle of this plant produces a marked action on the liver, causing jaundice.

Eyes.   Yellow discolouration. Swollen appearance.

Alimentary System.   The gums become spongy with a tendency to bleeding. Saliva is viscid. Hepatitis may develop leading to jaundice. Production of bile is impaired.

Renal System.   The urine becomes yellow and frothy and may contain urates and bile salts.

USES

Mainly of use in the treatment of sluggish liver action seen by jaundice and associated symptoms of yellowish urine and impaired digestion. Could be valuable in the treatment of kidney ailments which have their origin in the liver. Abundance of thick mucus in the throat.

Naja Tripudians

Cobra Venom.   The Ø is prepared from fresh poison in alcohol.

This poison produces a bulbar paralysis. Haemorrhages are scanty, but oedema is marked. The underlying tissues appear dark purple after the animal is bitten, blood-stained fluid being present in large quantities. Loss of limb control supervenes. Heart and lungs are also affected.

Eyes.   Heaviness of eyelids accompanies a fixed staring expression.

Ears.   Chronic discharges of blackish material.

Respiratory System.   A dry cough develops with difficult breathing.

Cardiac System.   Irregular tremulous pulse. Acute and chronic endocarditis may be seen according to the severity and duration of symptoms. Blood-pressure is lowered.

USES

May be employed in canine practice especially where general weakness in old animals accompanies heart trouble with associated dry coughing and palpitation. It may be of use in chronic ear canker, and in some cases of angio-neurotic oedema.

Natrum Arsenicum

Sodium Arsenate.   The Ø is prepared from trituration of salt.

Nasal catarrh is mainly associated with this salt. There may also be involvement of skin.

Respiratory System.   Nasal discharges producing crusty deposits. Cough accompanies a greenish expectoration.

Eyes.   Inflammation and agglutination of eyelids may develop into conjunctivitis. Oedema of lower lids.

Alimentary System.   The throat becomes dark purple and oedematous.

Extremities.   Stiffness of joints is a common feature.

USES

Eye conditions in general may be helped, especially the orbital cellulitis and oedema which sometimes is seen in distemper. Pharyngitis could benefit especially if accompanied by oedema.

Natrum Carbonicum

Sodium Carbonate.   The Ø is prepared from trituration of salt.

In common with other sodium salts this one stimulates cellular activity and increases metabolism, its action being more pronounced in the young animal.

Respiratory System.   Nasal discharge at first watery and later catarrhal.

Alimentary System.   There is a tendency to diarrhoea of young subjects especially if they are on a milk diet.

Extremities.   Weakness develops, the joints of the hind limb being especially affected.

Skin.   Vesicular eruptions may arise, the skin becoming dry, rough and cracked.

USES

This remedy may be of use in young calves where knuckling of fetlocks appears. It is also one of the remedies which helps control diarrhoea of milk origin. Exhausted and anaemic animals will usually show some response, especially those showing involvement of hind limb joints.

Natrum Muriaticum

Sodium Chloride.   The Ø is prepared from trituration of common salt.

Excessive intake of common salt leads to a condition of anaemia evidenced by dropsy or oedema of various parts. White blood cells are increased while mucous membranes are rendered dry.

Eyes.   Acrid lachrymation develops with swollen eyelids. Cataract may occur.

Respiratory System.   Thin, watery acrid nasal discharge arises. Difficult breathing develops with attendant cough.

Alimentary System.   Vesicles occur on the tongue accompanied by thirst. In the dog and cat there may be vomiting of whitish, glairy material. The appetite is usually indifferent and constipation is present.

Renal System.   Chronic nephritis develops over a long period, leading to the production of large amounts of clear urine of low specific gravity.

Extremities. Generalised weakness of limbs.

Skin. Various forms of eczema may develop accompanied by urticarial eruptions especially in bends of joints. Itching is usual. The hair may fall out in various body sites.

USES

This is a frequently used remedy which is of great value in chronic anaemic or unthrifty conditions. Salt retention leads to excessive thirst which may be seen in long-standing nephritic conditions of the dog and cat, and in these instances the infrequent use of high potencies usually gives good results. Its action on the skin makes it a useful remedy in eczema of debilitated subjects. Incipient cataract may respond along with generalised corneal opacities. It has been used successfully in periodic ophthalmia in the horse.

Natrum Salicylicum

Sodium Salicylate.   The Ø is prepared from trituration of the salt.

This salt produces an action on metabolism generally. The head, ears and kidneys are affected in particular.

Eyes. Affections of the iris are commonly produced. The retina may be the seat of haemorrhage.

Ears. Inflammation of the inner ear affects balance leading to vertigo.

Respiratory System. Difficult breathing with short sharp breath.

Skin. Urticarial swellings arise. Oedematous plaques may develop.

Alimentary System. The flow of bile is increased. Hepatitis sometimes arises.

Renal System. Chronic inflammation of the kidney develops. The urine may contain blood.

USES

Affections of the middle ear in small animals may find a use in this remedy, especially those accompanied by loss of balance. Sluggish liver conditions will be helped which in turn may lead to amelioration of kidney complaints. Angio-neurotic oedema suggests its use where other symptoms agree.

Natrum Sulphuricum

Sodium Sulphate.   The Ø is prepared from trituration of the salt.

Glauber's Salts produces a condition of weakness where the subject has been exposed to damp. The liver is affected and there is a tendency to wart formation.

Respiratory System. Nasal bleeding may occur, also thick, yellow catarrh. Difficult breathing develops, worse in damp weather.

Eyes. The conjunctiva becomes a dirty yellow colour.

Alimentary System. Hepatitis may arise with attendant jaundice. In the dog and cat vomiting of bilious material occurs. There is a tenderness over the liver region with flatulent distension and watery diarrhoea.

Renal System. The urine becomes loaded with bile-salts producing a reddish sediment. There is a tendency to the production of sugar in the urine.

Extremities. Lymphatic glandular swellings are seen together with oedema of lower limbs.

USES

Experience has proved this remedy to be of great value where there has been a history of head injury leading to a variety of seemingly unrelated conditions. The action on the liver makes it one of the remedies to be considered in hepatitis and jaundiced states. Diabetes in the dog could be favourably influenced.

Nitricum Acidum

Nitric Acid.   The Ø is prepared from solution in distilled water.

This acid affects particularly body outlets where mucous membrane and skin meet. It produces blisters and ulcers in the mouth and causes offensive discharges.

Eyes. Corneal ulceration develops. Acrid tears.

Respiratory System. Acrid nasal discharge leading to nose bleeding. Cough accompanies excoriating expectoration.

Alimentary System. Salivation together with bleeding gums. Tenderness develops over the region of the liver suggesting inflammation of that organ. Jaundice occurs with sometimes dysenteric, slimy stools.

Renal System. The urine is scanty, dark and strong-smelling. It may contain large amounts of albumen and casts.

Skin. Jagged warts develop which bleed easily. Granulations heal with difficulty.

USES

This remedy has a variety of uses in the older dog where warts develop accompanied by liver and kidney complaints. The action on mucocutaneous surfaces should not be forgotten as it is frequently these sites which are the seat of ulceration. Rodent ulcer may be helped, while in calves it has proved of value in some forms of mucosal disease.

Nux Moschata

Nutmeg. *N.O.* Myristicaceae. The Ø is prepared from powdered seeds.

This nut produces a fainting condition dependent on heart weakness or failure.

Respiratory System. Nasal bleeding, the blood being dark.

Alimentary System. The mouth is usually dry. The abdomen becomes bloated with flatulence.

Cardiac System. The pulse is weak and tremulous. There is a tendency to heart weakness with fainting spells.

Extremities. Pain is evident on handling the hindlimbs, especially the right, around hip and stifle, which is worse on movement.

USES

This remedy may be useful in rheumatic conditions of old dogs, especially if accompanied by heart weakness.

Nux Vomica

Poison Nut. *N.O.* Loganiaceae. The Ø is prepared from trituration of seeds.

Digestive disturbances and congestions are associated with this substance.

Eyes. Weakness of ocular muscles, leading to paresis.

Alimentary System. Flatulence and indigestion commonly occur. In the dog and cat vomiting takes place. There is tenderness over the stomach while the liver region is also sensitive to touch. Stools are generally hard.

Renal System. The urine is scanty and frequently contains blood.

Respiratory System. Shallow difficult breathing.

Extremities. Weakness develops over the lumbar region, with dragging gait.

USES

This is a useful remedy in abdominal and digestive disorders. Colic in the horse associated with ingestion of green food is one of the main indications for its use in that species. In sluggish digestive conditions it is sometimes combined with carbo vegetabilis in the form of carbo-nux. It has proved of value in the treatment of umbilical hernia of young subjects. Because of its action on the alimentary tract it is frequently prescribed as a preliminary remedy in cases of poisoning by certain plants which are capable of producing abdominal symptoms.

Ocimum Canum

N.O. Labiatae.   The Ø is prepared from the fresh leaves.

This is mainly a kidney remedy producing a variety of symptoms with an action on the renal system.

Alimentary System.   Tendency to frequent attacks of diarrhoea.

Renal System.   The urine becomes turbid and assumes a deep yellow colour. The urine may also become slimy and purulent with a musky smell. Reddish urine also occurs with a brick-dust-like sediment.

Female Genital System.   Swelling of the mammary glands.

USES

In veterinary practice used almost entirely in renal conditions which produce urine of the typical odour and appearance.

Opium

Dried Latex of Poppy.   *N.O.* Papaveraceae.   The Ø is prepared from tincture of exudation of capsule.

Opium produces an insensibility of the nervous system with stupor and torpor. There is a lack of vital reaction. All complaints are characterised by soporific states.

Head.   Dizzines and lack of balance, seen mostly in old subjects.

Eyes.   Pupils are contracted. The eyes assume a staring look.

Face.   Spasmodic twitching develops, especially near corners of the mouth. There is a tendency for the lower jaw to drop.

Alimentary System.   There is a blackish discolouration of the tongue which may also become paralysed. In the dog and cat there may be vomiting with convulsions. Appetite is lost. The abdomen is tympanitic with attendant constipation which may be extreme. Stools are generally black.

Renal System.   Urination is slow, difficult and may be painful.

Respiratory System.   Breathing becomes more stertorous accompanied sometimes by coughing.

Extremities.   There is a general paralysis, with a tendency to arching of the back. Twitching of muscles occurs.

USES

This remedy may be of benefit in severe cases of bowel inactivity associated with torpor or soporific states. It has been found in practice to be of great value in the treatment of conditions which have developed as a result of severe fright or shock.

Ornithogalum

Star of Bethlehem.   *N.O.* Liliaceae.   The Ø is prepared from fresh plant.

The active principle of this plant produces a marked action on the pylorus causing constriction with duodenal distension.

Alimentary System.   The tongue is coated. Flatulence develops with lack of appetite. There may be haemorrhage from the stomach with vomition in the dog and cat.

USES

This remedy may benefit chronic stomach complaints, especially in dogs where pyloric stenosis is suspected or confirmed. Affections of the duodenum may also improve under its use.

Osmium

The Element.   The Ø is prepared from trituration of metal.

Osmium produces an effect on the respiratory and cutaneous systems, with an action also on structures of the eye.

Eyes.   There is an increase in tension in the chambers of the eye. This leads to glaucoma which is a common development. There is aversion to light accompanying a conjunctivitis.

Respiratory System.   The larynx becomes inflamed leading to a throaty cough, accompanied by stringy mucous discharge.

Skin.   Eczema develops with production of itching pimply rash.

USES

This remedy is worth considering in the treatment of glaucoma in the dog. If given early it may possibly arrest the condition and keep it manageable. Inflammatory conditions of the larynx may also benefit.

Oxytropis

Loco Weed.   *N.O.* Leguminosae.   The Ø is prepared from fresh plant.

The nervous system is markedly affected by this plant. There is a tendency to walk backwards.

Eyes.   Pupils become contracted. Paralysis of nerves and muscles of eye.

Extremities.   Loss of co-ordination develops. The muscles become stiff.

USES

This is one of the remedies that should be considered in the treatment of cerebro-cortical necrosis of sheep and cattle. It could also supplement other remedies in cases of swayback and louping-ill.

Palladium

The Metal.   The Ø is prepared from trituration of metal.

This element produces its main action on the female genital system, especially the ovary, causing an inflammation with a tendency to uterine prolapse and pelvic peritonitis.

USES

Ovarian dysfunction of cows and heifers comes within its sphere of action. It may therefore benefit irregularities of the oestrus cycle when dependent on ovarian under-activity. Also in cystic ovary. Pelvic disorders dependent on ovaritis should also benefit, especially on the right side.

Petroleum

Rock Spirit.   The Ø is prepared from the oil.

This spirit produces cutáneous eruptions and catarrh of mucous membranes.

Eyes.   A dry scurfy rash develops around the eyelids.

Ears.   Chronic middle ear catarrh. Eczema of ear flaps. Fissures inside ear.

Respiratory System.   Bleeding from ulcerated nostrils. Difficult breathing.

Skin.   Blistery eruptions. Dry skin. Generalised eczema.

USES

Mainly used as an eczema remedy in small animal practice. Specific areas around eyes and ears may determine its use in preference to other seemingly indicated remedies. Complaints are usually worse in winter.

Phaseolus

Dwarf Bean.   *N.O.* Leguminoseae.   The Ø is prepared from trituration of dried bean.

This substance produces a marked action on the heart.

Respiratory System. Breathing is slowed. Pleurisy may develop.

Cardiac System. Effusions occur into the pericardial sac. Rapid pulse. Pain on pressure over cardiac area.

Renal System. The urine may become diabetic.

Eyes. Aversion to light. Pressure on eyeballs is resented. Dilation of pupils.

USES

Old dogs with heart complaints and a tendency to diabetes may benefit. Secondary pleurisy with effusions come within the sphere of action.

Phosphoricum Acidum

Phosphoric Acid. The Ø is prepared from dilution in distilled water.

This acid produces a debilitating state in which flatulence and diarrhoea are common symptoms.

Respiratory System. Bleeding from nose. Difficult breathing with dry cough.

Alimentary System. Gums become swollen with production of viscid mucus and blood. The abdomen is distended and pale diarrhoea occurs.

Renal System. Urination is profuse. Urine contains phosphatic deposits.

Cardiac System. Rapid irregular pulse.

Extremities. Weakness of all limbs.

Skin. Pimply eruptions alternate with blood-filled blisters. Ulcers may arise with tendency to pus formation.

USES

This remedy may be of use in interdigital cyst in the dog, where the lesion takes the form of blood-blister. Diabetes insipidus may benefit. It has some value in helping metabolism in the young rapidly growing dog.

Phosphorus

The Element. The Ø is prepared from trituration of red phosphorus.

This important substance produces an inflammatory and degenerative effect on mucous membranes and causes bone destruction and necrosis of liver.

Eyes. Degenerative changes occur in the retinal cells. The conjunctivae are invariably pale. The eyelids are oedematous while cataract and glaucoma are frequent complications.

Respiratory System. Periostitis of nasal bones produces bleeding with catarrhal inflammation. Difficult breathing with hard dry cough. Pneumonia is common with extensive hepatisation leading to rust-coloured expectoration.

Alimentary System. The gums become ulcerated and bloody. Thirst is present but vomition takes place in the dog and cat shortly after taking food or water. Tenderness is common over the stomach region. Signs of abdominal colic appear. The liver becomes congested with hepatitis, jaundice and pancreatic disease common sequelae. Stools are pale and clay-coloured.

Renal System. The urine is brown and turbid and may contain blood with a reddish sediment occurring.

Cardiac System. Weak rapid pulse.

Extremities. There is frequently an ascending paralysis of sensory and motor nerves with trembling of muscles.

Skin. Small punctiform haemorrhages arise which heal and tend to break out again. Purpura-like states with jaundice.

USES

This is a very important remedy and has proved its worth in a great variety of conditions met with in veterinary practice. Among these may be mentioned pneumonia of rapid onset in all species. Progressive retinal atrophy in the dog: Hepatitis and periostitis: cataract and glaucoma. In gastritis of dogs and cats a guiding symptom is vomition of stomach contents as soon as they become warm, shortly after ingestion. Superficial small haemorrhages also respond.

Physostigma

Calabar Bean. *N.O.* Leguminoseae. The Ø is prepared from trituration of bean.

The active principle of this plant increases peristalsis and raises the heart rate and blood-pressure.

Head. Spastic conditions of facial muscles develop.

Eyes. The pupils are contracted, with twitching of ocular muscles. Profuse lachrymation occurs and glaucoma may develop.

Respiratory System. Nasal discharges occur leading to herpetic eruptions around the nostrils.

Cardiac System. Pronounced heart beat. Jugular pulse may be seen.

Extremities. Muscular cramps and tetanic seizures are common.

USES

Has been used effectivly in some forms of epileptic seizures in dogs. There is usually an accompanying diarrhoea and eye involvement when it is indicated.

Phytolacca

Poke Root. *N.O.* Phytolaccaceae. The Ø is prepared from whole fresh plant.

A state of restlessness and prostration is associated with this plant, together with glandular swellings.

Eyes. Increased lachrymal discharge.

Respiratory System. One-sided nasal discharge. Dry cough.

Alimentary System. Throat involvement takes the form of dark red discolouration with swelling of tonsillar tissue, making swallowing difficult. Parotid glands become swollen and tender.

Renal System. Nephritis with scanty urine.

Female Genital System. Mammary glands become hard and painful. Tumours may develop. Abscess formation is common as is mastitis in various forms. Milk flow is increased.

Male Genital System. Swelling of testicles occurs.

Skin. Papular and pustular eruptions may develop into boil formation. Various forms of eczema may be seen.

USES

This remedy is of great value in mastitis of cattle where it can profitably be combined with other remedies. It has been used successfully in both acute and chronic forms. It will help arrest the growth of mammary tumours in the bitch if given early. Glandular swellings in general are benefited. It is a remarkably good remedy for sore throats, pharyngitis and parotid swellings.

Picricum Acidum

Picric Acid. The Ø is prepared from solution in rectified spirit.

This acid produces a state of anaemia with kidney involvement. It also acts on the sexual organs.

Eyes. Chronic catarrhal conjunctivitis occurs with copious yellow discharge.

Renal System. Nephritis. Urine may be suppressed with a uraemic tendency. The urine contains casts and is dark and blood-stained.

Male Genital System. There is a tendency to hypertrophy of the prostate gland. Sexual desire may be increased.

Female Genital System. Discharge occurs from the uterus.

USES

This remedy may be of use in the treatment of old male dogs showing prostatic enlargement. Certain types of kidney disease will also benefit more especially in the older animal. Associated eye symptoms may provide a clue to its use.

Pilocarpus

Jaborandi. Pilocarpinum. The Ø is prepared from solution of the alkaloid in distilled water.

The active principle produces increased salivation and sweat formation. Lachyrmal secretions are also increased.

Eyes. Contraction of pupils. Twitching of eyelids.

Alimentary System. Copious salivation. Profuse diarrhoea with straining. Sub-maxillary and parotid salivary glands become swollen.

Renal System. Only a small amount of urine passed at any one time.

Cardiac System. Cyanosis. Irregular pain.

Respiratory System. Difficult breathing. Bronchitis. Oedema of lungs.

Skin. Excessive perspiration. Dry patchy eczema.

USES

A useful remedy where excessive salivation is associated with swelling of parotid glands. Conditions which accompany profuse sweating in the horse may respond well.

Platina

Platinum. The Ø is prepared from trituration with lactose.

This metal has a specific action on the female genital system, especially the ovaries where inflammation readily develops and the production of cysts is not uncommon.

USES

A useful remedy for controlling irregular heat periods especially where the ovary function is disturbed.

Plumbum Metallicum

Lead.   The Ø is prepared from trituration with lactose.

A state of paralysis preceded by pain is produced by metallic lead. It affects the central nervous system and also causes jaundice and anaemia.

Head.   Delirium and convulsions leading to coma.

Eyes.   Contraction of pupils. Purulent conjunctivitis leading to glaucoma. Eyes may have a yellowish discolouration.

Alimentary System.   Gums become swollen and may have a bluish look. There is paralysis of tongue leading to an inability to swallow solids. Colicky pains develop. Stools become dark and hard. There is a tendency to hernia.

Renal System.   Difficulty in passing urine which is albuminous. Chronic kidney degeneration. Cystitis.

Cardiac System.   Weakness of heart action producing a small irregular pulse.

Extremities.   Paralysis of lower limbs develops.

Skin.   Jaundiced appearance with dryness.

USES

This is an important remedy to be considered in chronic degenerative kidney disease with possible liver involvement. Convulsive states may benefit from its use along with various forms of paralysis, e.g. radial in the horse. The paralytic action suggests that it could be worth trying in grass sickness in the horse, particularly the sub-acute form with colic and muscular weakness and atrophy.

Podophyllum

May Apple.   *N.O.* Ranunculaceae.   The Ø is prepared from whole fresh plant.

The active principle of this plant exerts is action mainly on the duodenum and small intestine causing an enteritis. The liver and rectum are also affected.

Alimentary System.   In the dog and cat vomiting occurs. There is thirst for very cold water. Distension of abdomen is seen with a tendency to lie on the belly. Colicky pains develop with tenderness over the liver area. A watery greenish diarrhoea may alternate with constipation.

USES

This may be a useful remedy in gastro-intestinal disorders of young
animals especially, e.g. during dentition. May be indicated in cases of
liver engorgement and portal congestion with jaundice. In post-partum
conditions of the bitch associated with straining and abdominal discomfort it could also be of value.

Populus Tremuloides

American Aspen. *N.O.* Solicaceae. The Ø is prepared from the
inner bark.

Gastric and urinary disorders leading to anorexia and weakness are
associated with this plant.

Alimentary System. Flatulence is common along with vomiting in the dog and cat.

Renal System. Straining to pass urine occurs. The urine is
purulent. In the male prostatic enlargement develops.

USES

Mainly used in the various kidney and bladder complaints of old dogs
especially those showing an associated prostate enlargement.

Prunus Spinosa

Blackthorn. *N.O.* Rosaceae. The Ø is prepared from buds before
flowering.

This plant produces a marked action on the urinary organs and
extremities.

Alimentary System. Ascites develops.

Renal System. Weakness of bladder musculature produces
straining to pass urine.

Respiratory System. Wheezing respiration occurs.

Skin. Herpetic eruptions develop.

Extremities. Oedema of lower limbs.

USES

Its special action on the kidneys determines its use in certain forms of
nephritis leading to oedema.

Psorinum

Scabies Vesicle. The Ø is prepared from trituration of dried vesicle.

This nosode produces a state of debility, especially after acute illness, with skin symptoms predominating. All discharges are unpleasant.

Eyes. Inflammation of lids which become agglutinated. Chronic ophthalmia.

Alimentary System. Ulcerated gums. Swollen throat. Abdominal pain.

Respiratory System. Chronic nasal discharge. Hard dry cough.

Ears. Otitis media and externa. Brownish discharge.

Extremities. Eruptions around nails. Joint weakness.

Skin. Dry coat. Offensive eczema. Herpetic eruptions with severe itch.

USES

Of value in eczematous conditions where well-chosen remedies fail to act. Skin conditions are accompanied by a musty smell. Should not be used in low potency or repeated too often. Could prove of value in ear canker with foul-smelling discharge. Animals needing psorinum generally seek warmth.

Ptelea

Wafer Ash. *N.O.* Rutaceae. The Ø is prepared from bark of root.

This plant produces an action on stomach and liver.

Alimentary System. Excessive salivation. Papillae of tongue red and prominent. Vomiting in the dog and cat. Hepatitis with tenderness over liver and stomach regions.

Respiratory System. Difficult breathing.

USES

Of use in liver and abdominal affections, e.g. portal congestions. Should be remembered if other commoner remedies fail to act.

Pulsatilla

Anemone. *N.O.* Ranunculaceae. The Ø is prepared from whole fresh plant.

Mucous membranes in general come within the sphere of action of this plant.

Ears. Thick bland discharges.

Eyes. Catarrhal discharges. Lachrymation. Inflamed lids.

Respiratory System. Nasal discharge. Bland expectorations.

Renal System. Increased urination.

Female Genital System. Uterine discharge of bland catarrhal or mucus material. Ovarian hypofunction.

Male Genital System.   Inflammation of testicles and prostate gland.

Skin.   Urticarial eczema.

USES

A useful remedy for the bitch showing a tendency to pyometra and false pregnancy. Has been used successfully for retained placenta in cattle. Feline influenza with typical eye symptoms should respond to its use. The action on the ovary suggests its use in the treatment of ovarian under-activity leading to infertility.

Pyrogenium

Artificial Sepsin.   The Ø is prepared from solutions in water (distilled).

This nosode has a specific relation to septic inflammations associated with offensive discharges.

Alimentary System.   In the dog and cat there may be vomiting of dark material, offensive diarrhoea with straining. May be blood-stained.

Cardiac System.   Weak thready pulse is the rule, but occasionally there may be a bounding tense pulse.

Female Genital System.   Puerperal feverish states, especially associated with abortion or miscarriage. Post-partum bleeding.

Skin.   Small wounds tend to become septic quickly.

USES

This is a very valuable remedy in certain septic conditions where, e.g. usually a high temperature accompanies a thready, weak pulse. It should always be given in frequent repetition after abortion in cattle where its early use may help prevent retention of afterbirth.

Radium

Radium Bromide.   The Ø is prepared from trituration of the salt.

The bromide of this element is the salt usually employed. It produces a state of general weakness and debility with pains in various parts.

Alimentary System.   Tympanitic cramp with rumbling of gas. Generally a loose stool.

Renal System. Increased elimination of solids, especially chlorides. Nephritis with albuminuria and casts in the urine.

Respiratory System.   Dry cough with laryngitis.

Extremities.   Painful joints which may develop into arthritis especially of carpus and tarsus.

Skin.   Erythema. Dermatitis of feet. Itching and swelling.

USES

This remedy may be of value in arthritic conditions of dogs with an associated nephritis. Could be worth trying in cases of generalised debility and weakness.

Ranunculus Bulbosus

Buttercup.   *N.O.* Ranunculaceae.   The Ø is prepared from whole plant.

The action is mainly on muscular tissue and skin producing a hyper-sensibility to touch.

Eyes.   Herpetic vesicles on cornea with lachrymation.

Respiratory System.   Pain over intercostal region.

Skin.   Intense itching. Herpetic vesicular eruptions. Blister-like eruptions on feet, frequently bluish and clustering together in oval-shaped groups.

USES

A good remedy in certain types of eczema showing the typical rash rheumatism of intercostal region.

Rhamnus Californica

Californian Poppy.   *N.O.* Rhamnaceae.   The Ø is prepared from ripe berries.

A rheumatic-like condition of muscles and joints is associated with this plant.

Respiratory System.   Tenderness over intercostal muscles.

Extremities.   Pain and tenderness in muscles and joints.

USES

Mainly of use in rheumatic-like conditions.

Rheum

Rhubarb.   *N.O.* Polygonaceae.   The Ø is prepared from trituration of dried root.

Rhubarb produces a sour-smelling diarrhoea, especially in young subjects.

Alimentary System.   Difficult teething. Sour-smelling breath. Colicky pains precede diarrhoea with shivering and straining.

USES

This remedy could be of value in abdominal complaints associated with teething. Also in coli-bacillosis and associated complaints in calves and lambs where the resulting diarrhoea has the typically sour smell.

Rhododendron

Snow Rose.   *N.O.* Ericaceae.   The Ø is prepared from fresh leaves.

This shrub causes rheumatic-like or gouty symptoms, more especially in humid weather.

Male Genital System.   Swelling of testicles with a tendency to induration.

Extremities.   Joints become swollen. Gouty inflammation of toes. Stiffness of neck.

USES

This remedy may be of use in testicular swellings, occasionally seen in the ram. Conditions simulating rheumatism in old dogs may also benefit.

Rhus Aromatica

Fragrant Sumach. *N.O.* Anacardaceae. The Ø is prepared from fresh root bark.

The active principle acts mainly on kidney and bladder.

Renal System.   The urine becomes albuminous and may contain blood. There is a tendency to diabetes with urine of a low specific gravity. Cystitis develops with the presence of a weak bladder musculature. The animal may exhibit signs of pain before urinating and incontinence may develop.

USES

This remedy should be considered in old dogs and cats which present symptoms of bladder weakness and/or nephritis, especially of a chronic nature. It may also prove useful in diabetes.

Rhus Toxicodendron

Poison Ivy. *N.O.* Anacardaceae. The Ø is prepared from fresh leaves before flowering.

The active principles of this tree affect skin and muscles together with mucous membranes and fibrous tissues producing tearing pains and blistery eruptions.

Eyes.   Orbital cellulitis develops, the eyelids being red and swollen. Pustules may arise on the cornea. Oedema of eyelids which become swollen and agglutinated.

Ears.   Inflammation of inner and outer ear. Discharges may be blood-stained. The left ear is more often affected.

Respiratory System.   Nasal discharge which may contain blood. Bleeding from lungs may take place.

Head and Face.   Swollen appearance. Inflammation of parotid glands, especially the left.

Alimentary System.   Tongue and throat dark red and inflamed. Thirst is present. Dysentery with mucus.

Renal System.   The urine is dark and scanty with a whitish sediment on standing.

Female Genital System.   Offensive dark, uterine discharges.

Cardiac System.   Weak intermittent pulse.

Extremities.   Stiffness of joints and muscles arises. This is alleviated on moving.

Skin.   A red erysipeloid rash develops accompanied by vesicles and urticarial swellings. Superficial glands become swollen. Cellulitis is a common feature.

USES

This is a very useful remedy for various conditions met with in veterinary practice. It is indicated in many spheres, e.g. the eye lesions of distemper accompanied by orbital cellulitis. Also in rheumatic states and in skin rashes showing erythema and vesicular swellings. Tendon sprains of horses may respond well and in this connection it could also be employed externally in the form of a liniment. A guiding symptom to the employment of this remedy is that the animal usually shows improvement on moving.

Rhus Venenata

Poison Elder. *N.O.* Anacardaceae. The Ø is prepared from fresh leaves and stem.

This shrub produces an action similar to Rhus toxicodendron, but the skin symptoms are more severe.

Ears. Vesicular inflammation.
Eyes. Severe swelling of eyelids.
Skin. Itching vesicles. Inflammation very acute. Skin appears dark red.

USES

This remedy may produce good results in the more severe vesicular eczemas where Rhus toxicodendron appears to be indicated but fails to produce relief.

Rumex Crispus

Yellow Dock. *N.O.* Polygonaceae. The Ø is prepared from fresh root.

Pains varying in severity and distribution are associated with this plant. It is capable of diminishing the secretions of mucous membranes.

Alimentary System. Chronic gastritis. Aversion to food. Watery diarrhoea.

Respiratory System. Mucous discharges take place from trachea and nose. These tend to be frothy.

Skin. Intense urticarial itching especially of the lower limbs.

USES

This is a useful remedy in certain respiratory conditions and also in cases of lymphatic vessel enlargement.

Ruta Graveolens

Rue.   *N.O.* Rutaceae.   The Ø is prepared from whole fresh plant.

Ruta produces its action on the periosteum and cartilages with an action also on eyes and uterus. Deposits arise around the carpal joints under its use.

Eyes.   Redness with aversion to light.

Renal System.   There is urging to urinate.

Alimentary System.   Various affections of the lower bowel are seen. There is frequent discharge of blood at stool.

Respiratory System.   Coughing with yellowish expectoration.

Extremities.   Weakness of back and legs when first moving. Tendinitis and periostitis may arise.

USES

In veterinary practice it has a proven use in the treatment of tendon weakness and inflammations of periosteal surfaces. It is of use in conditions affecting the lower rectum and may help reduce rectal prolapse. It is a useful eye remedy.

Sabina

Savine. *N.O.* Coniferae. The Ø is prepared from the oil or from young branches.

The uterus is the main seat of the action of this plant. It produces a tendency to abortion. There is also an action on fibrous tissues and serous membranes. It is associated with haemorrhages of bright red blood which remains fluid.

Renal System. Inflammation of bladder and urethra causing blood to appear in urine.

Female Genital System. Threatened abortion with discharge of blood. There is a lack of tone in the uterine muscle. Inflammation of ovaries.

USES

This remedy has its main use in uterine conditions including retained placenta. Also in pyometra associated with much blood. Post-partum haemorrhage will be alleviated in uncomplicated non-septic states.

Salicylicum Acidum

Salicylic Acid. The Ø is prepared from trituration of dried acid.

This acid produces rheumatic-like states and dyspepsia. Also ulceration of mucous and serous membranes.

Eyes. Haemorrhages develop on the retina.

Alimentary System. Inflammation of the throat causing difficulty in swallowing. Putrid diarrhoea results from gastro-enteritis. The faeces are greenish.

Extremities. Joints become swollen.

Skin. Vesicular eruptions arise with urticaria, purpura and herpes.

USES

It has its main use in articular affections, especially rheumatic-like conditions of small joints. Canker sores in the mouth may be helped.

Pharyngitis and stomatitis should also be alleviated. Its action on the skin should not be overlooked and it may be useful in various eczematous conditions associated with purpura-like swellings.

Sanguinaria

Blood Root.   *N.O.* Papaveraceae.   The Ø is prepared from fresh root.
An alkaloid sanguinarine contained in this plant has an affinity with the circulatory system, leading to congestion and redness.
Female Genital System.   Bleeding from uterus. Inflammation of ovaries.
Alimentary System.   Gastro-enteritis. Mucous membranes become dry.
Extremities.   Stiffness of fore-legs especially left shoulder region.
Circulatory System.   Congestion of blood-vessles. Small cutaneous haemorrhages arise in various sites.
Eyes.   Red appearance. Inflammation of the conjunctiva.

USES
Has its main use in conditions associated with congestions of blood-vessels, especially those of the respiratory tract and skin.

Sambucus Nigra

Elder.   *N.O.* Capufoliacea.   The Ø is prepared from fresh leaves and flowers.
The action of the active principle of this tree is chiefly on the respiratory system.
Renal System.   Frequent urination. Large amounts of urine passed. Acute nephritis with associated dropsical conditions.
Extremities.   Various types of oedematous swelling develop.
Respiratory System.   Accumulation of mucus in the larynx may impede normal respiration. Coughing develops.
Skin.   Oedematous swellings arise.

USES
Affections of the kidney and respiratory tract come within its sphere of action.

Santoninum

Santonine.   The Ø is prepared from trituration and subsequent dilution in alcohol.

This substance has a specific action on the alimentary tract where it sets up vomiting and purging. The kidneys and bladder are also markedly affected.

Eyes. Pupils distorted. Fixed staring look. Pupils widely dilated. Photophobia and lachrymation.

Head. Convulsive twitching of face muscles. Lips drawn over teeth, and severely swollen.

Alimentary System. Tongue red and dry. Frothing at mouth. Swelling of parotid and submaxillary glands. Lack of appetite. Great thirst. Rumbling in abdomen preceding violent diarrhoea.

Renal System. Urination difficult. Urine deep yellow. Haemoglobinuria. Cystitis.

Extremities. Twitching of limbs. Convulsive jerking. Staggering gait.

USES

Because of its action on the intestines this remedy has a good reputation as an anthelmintic. A guiding symptom to its use in urinary distrubances is the saffron colour of the urine.

Scrophularia Nodosa

Figwort. *N.O.* Scrophulaneceae. The Ø is prepared from whole fresh plant.

Exerts its main action on the lymphatic system and skin.

Ears. Eczema appears on the outer skin. There may be ulceration within the ear flap.

Alimentary System. There is slight inflammatory action on the liver giving rise to tenderness over the hepatic region.

Female Genital System. Small tumours and nodosities appear in the mammary glands.

Lymphatic System. Lymphatic glands become swollen.

USES

This is a useful remedy in treatment of mammary tumours in the bitch. Lymphadenitis may also respond to its use, while its action on the ear suggests its use in some forms of ear canker.

Scutellaria Lateriflora

Skull Cap. *N.O.* Labiatae. The Ø is prepared from the fresh plant.

This plant exerts its main influence on the central nervous system which determines its main use. Excitable and hysterical states are common.

Alimentary System. Vomiting. Poor appetite. Colic.

Central Nervous System. Vertigo. Photophobia. Hysteria convulsions.

USES
Used mainly as one of the remedies likely to be of use in hysterical states of excitable dogs.

Secale Cornutum

Ergot of Rye. *N.O.* Fungi. The Ø is prepared from fresh fungus.

Ergot is a fungus which produces marked contraction of smooth muscle, causing a diminution of blood-supply to various areas. This is particularly seen in peripheral blood-vessels especially of the feet.

Eyes. Incipient cataract. Eyes become sunken.

Alimentary System. Great thirst. In the dog and cat vomiting of blood may arise. Stools are dark green alternating with dysentery.

Respiratory System. Difficulty in breathing.

Female Genital System. Bleeding from uterus with putrid discharges.

Extremities. Cold feet and legs, due to impaired circulation. Muscular trembling sometimes seen.

Skin. There is tendency to gangrene with a shrivelled dry appearance. Ulcerations develop with bleeding from cutaneous vessels. Dark red livid areas sometimes seen.

USES
Because of its circulatory action and effect on unstriped muscle it is useful in many uterine conditions, e.g. pyometra and post-partum haemorrhages with dark blood. It has been used with success in some forms of interdigital cyst and foot swellings in the dog, where blood-blisters and livid cysts develop. This remedy will aid normal circulation in the feet of animals trapped by wire snares if given in time.

Selenium

The Element. The Ø is prepared from trituration with lactose.

The chief action of this metal is on the genito-urinary system. The skin is also affected to a lesser degree.

Alimentary System.   Tenderness over liver region. Hepatitis may develop. The enlarged liver may be palpated readily.

Renal System.   Weakness of bladder muscles leads to a loss of power to expel urine.

Male Genital System.   The prostate gland is affected giving rise to swelling which compounds the difficulty in passing urine.

Skin.   Dryness and pruritus develop, especially on feet and toes. The hair may fall out and vesicular eruptions sometimes arise.

USES
Could prove useful in the treatment of genito-urinary conditions of old male dogs, e.g. prostatic hypertrophy with skin involvement. Various forms of eczema in the cat and dog may respond well.

Sempervivum Tectorum

House Leek.   *N.O.* Crassulaceae.   The Ø is prepared from fresh leaves.

The main affinity of this plant is with skin and connective tissue giving rise to herpetic eruptions and tumour formation.

Alimentary System.   Tumours develop around and in the mouth with ulceration.

Skin.   Erysipeloid affections. Warty growths may arise.

USES
Mammary tumours in the bitch may be relieved by this remedy. Has been used successfully in various eczematous and other skin affections, e.g. ringworm and wart formation. It should therefore be remembered as a remedy worth trying for these conditions where more commonly used remedies fail to alleviate.

Senecio Aureus

Ragwort.   *N.O.* Compositae.   The Ø is prepared from fresh plant in flower.

This species of ragwort produces action on the kidneys and on the female genital system.

Alimentary System.   The liver becomes cirrhosed, giving rise to an involvement of the portal circulation which leads to a dysenteric stool. There is tenderness over the liver area.

Renal System.   Nephritis develops which may be manifested by blood in the urine and difficulty in urination.

Female Genital System.   Congestive states within the uterus lead to discharges which may be muco-purulent and blood-stained.

Respiratory System.   Acute inflammatory conditions of the upper tract develop leading to a loose congestive cough.

USES

This remedy could have some value in congestive liver conditions and early cirrhotic states. It is also one of the many remedies which may be indicated in nephritis of the dog particularly.

Sepia

Ink of the Cuttlefish.   The Ø is prepared from dried liquid.

Portal congestion and stasis are associated with this substance along with disturbances of function in the female genital system.

Eyes.   Congestion of venous blood-vessels.

Ears.   Herpetic eruptions develop behind the ears with swelling.

Alimentary System.   Lack of appetite with poor digestion. Tenderness occurs over liver.

Renal System.   Chronic cystitis is commonly seen. Urine may be reddish and contains deposits.

Female Genital System.   Tenderness around pelvic area. Prolapse of uterus may occur. Various types of discharge arise.

Extremities.   The animal's hind legs may give out due to a weakness in the sacral region.

Skin.   Small itching spots arise with herpetic eruptions.

USES

This is a very useful remedy, used in a wide variety of conditions, but principally employed in the female where it has given good results in pyometra in the bitch and infertility of indeterminate cause in the larger animals. It has a use in some forms of skin affections such as alopecia and ringworm. Post-partum discharges are favourably influenced. It is capable of promoting the maternal instinct in those animals which are indifferent to their young.

Serum Anguillar Ichthyotoxin

Eel Serum.   The Ø is prepared from dried serum or solution in distilled water.

The serum of the eel produces an action on the blood equivalent to toxaemia. It affects the kidney particularly with secondary effects on the liver. Renal deposits are found in the urine along with haemoglobin.

Threatened uraemic states develop frequently. The cardiac system is
also affected, sudden fainting spells being common.

USES

This is a valuable remedy in anuria with threatened uraemia; also in
heart disease when diuresis is indicated and associated with kidney
failure. In sudden onset with threatened uraemia higher potencies
should be employed, e.g. 30c. The lower potencies, e.g. 3x – 6x should
be reserved for those animals showing heart symptoms.

Silicea

Flint.   The Ø is prepared from pure substance.

The main action of this substance is on bone where it is capable of
causing caries and necrosis. It also produces abscesses and fistulae of
connective tissue with fibrous growths.

Eyes.   Inflammation of the iris develops with suppurative tendency. The cornea is the seat of ulceration and abscess.

Alimentary System.   The parotid glands become inflamed.
Diarrhoea may alternate with constipation.

Glandular System.   The inguinal and cervical glands especially
become swollen.

Renal System.   Sediment appears in the urine which may be
blood-stained.

Female Genital System.   Hard swellings develop in the
mammary glands.

Respiratory System.   Various suppurative processes may arise
as the result of the general tendency to abscess formation, e.g. bron-
chiectasis.

Extremities.   Caries of spinal processes. Loss of power in legs.
Contraction of tendons.

Skin.   Abscesses and fistulae predominate. Ulcerations. Tumour
formation. There is a tendency for all wounds to suppurate.

USES

This is a widely used remedy, indicated in many suppurative processes
usually after acute symptoms have passed and a chronic state has arisen.
This is manifested by sinuses and fistulae where its use has given consistently good results. Certain forms of anaemia benefit from high
potencies infrequently repeated. It is a useful eye remedy where
corneal ulceration has developed. Specific conditions where it has been
employed to good effect include summer mastitis of cattle, poll-evil and
fistulous withers and sandcrack in the horse, interdigital cysts in the

dog and actinobacillosis of cattle. It is capable of causing regression of some forms of tumour and hastening the absorption of scar tissue.

Solidago Virga

Golden Rod. *N.O.* Compositae. The Ø is prepared from whole fresh plant.

This plant produces an inflammatory action on parenchymatous organs particularly the kidney.

Eyes. Increased secretion leading to burning discharges.

Respiratory System. Muco-purulent expectoration with cough.

Renal System. Scanty reddish urine with albuminuria.

Male Genital System. Enlargement of prostate may occur.

Skin. Exanthematous eruptions of lower limbs accompany the kidney symptoms.

USES

This remedy may be of use in acute renal insufficiency where diuresis is desired. It can produce results which obviate the use of the catheter, and also has some value in prostatic enlargement.

Spartium Scoparium

Broome. The main action is produced on the heart, slowing the action and reducing blood-pressure. It acts directly on the myocardium weakening the contractions, and causes also an increase in urination.

Cardiac System. Irregular heart action. Degeneration of heart muscle.

Renal System. Nephritis with increase in the amount of urine passed.

USES

This is a useful remedy in promoting diuresis in dropsical states which are dependent on weak heart action, and is therefore of use in canine practice for treatment of older dogs which frequently are presented with symptoms of failing heart.

Spigelia

Pink Root. *N.O.* Loganaceae. The Ø is prepared from dried herb.

Has an affinity for the nervous system and also exerts an action on the cardiac region and the eye.

Eyes.   Pupils usually dilated. Ophthalmia frequently arises.

Cardiac System.   Irregular pulse. Palpitation and shortness of breath, worse on movement.

USES

This could be a useful remedy in pericarditis, while other heart conditions giving discomfort on movement may be helped. The action on eye structures should not be overlooked.

Spongia Tosta

Roasted Sponge.   The Ø is prepared from solution in alcohol.

The sponge produces symptoms related to the respiratory and cardiac spheres. The lymphatic system is also affected.

Eyes.   Watery or mucous discharges.

Alimentary System.   Vesicular eruptions develop on tongue and gums. Dryness of throat with excessive hunger and thirst.

Glandular System.   Enlargement of thyroid gland. Swollen indurated lymphatic glands.

Male Genital System.   Swelling of testicles.

Respiratory System.   Dryness of mucous membranes of air passages producing a cough which tends to disappear on drinking.

Cardiac System.   Affections of heart valves leading mainly to insufficiency. Reflex coughing may be produced.

Skin.   Itching eruptions develop.

USES

This is a valuable remedy in small animal practice where it helps control the sympathetic coughing associated with heart disease. Orchitis in the ram has been successfully treated. The general action on glands suggests its use in lymphadenitis of varying origin while its specific action on the thyroid gland could be of value in cases of goitre occasionally seen in dogs.

Squilla Maritima

Sea Onion.   *N.O.* Liliaceae.   The Ø is prepared from dried bulb.

Acts especially on the mucous membranes of the respiratory tract. The digestive system and kidneys are also affected.

Respiratory System.   Nasal discharge. Dry cough which later becomes mucous.

Cardiac System. Fibrillation of heart muscle occurs.

Renal System. Urging to urinate, the urine being watery and profuse.

USES

This is a useful remedy for heart and kidney affections, being especially valuable in dropsical conditions.

Staphisagria

Stavesacre. *N.O.* Ranunculaceae. The Ø is prepared from seeds.

The nervous system is mainly involved, but there is also an action on the genito-urinary tract and the skin.

Eyes. Orbital eczema occurs along with inflammation of the cornea.

Alimentary System. Gums become swollen, bleeding easily. Salivation is accompanied by excessive hunger. The abdomen is swollen with evidence of colic.

Renal System. Frequent urination with urging after the bladder has been emptied. Cystitis in general.

Skin. Eczema of the head region including ears, producing thick scabs.

USES

This remedy may benefit some cases of cystitis, especially in the female subject. Skin symptoms accompanying the renal and nervous states are a useful guide to its selection. Its action on the eye has determined its use in tarsal growths and blepharitis. It is a useful post-operative remedy being able to restore tissues to normal in a short time, thus reducing the convalescent period.

Stigmata Maydis

Corn Silk. *N.O.* Gramineae. The Ø is prepared from solution in alcohol.

The urinary tract is chiefly involved.

Renal System. Retention of urine with difficulty in expulsion. The urine contains thick sediment, which may be blood-stained. Inflammation of bladder causing straining after urination.

USES

This is one of the many remedies which can be of value in cystitis promoting a normal flow of urine. It has thus a place in the treatment of ascites and oedematous states generally. Prostatic enlargement may also be helped.

Stramonium

Thorn Apple. *N.O.* Solanaceae. The Ø is prepared from whole fresh plant and fruit.

The active principle of this shrub produces its main action on the central nervous system, especially the cerebrum.

Head. Staggering gait dependent on brain involvement. There is a tendency to fall forward.

Eyes. Dilated pupils with a fixed, staring look.

Alimentary System. Viscid salivation producing a chewing motion.

Female Genital System. Bleeding from uterus. Puerperal convulsions.

Extremities. Chorea. Convulsive movements of upper limbs and isolated groups of muscles. Trembling and staggering gaits.

Central Nervous System. Epileptic type fits.

USES

This remedy has a role to play in helping control the brain symptoms of such conditions as hypomagnesaemia. It is also of use in lactation tetany in the bitch. Specific conditions which may benefit include cerebro-cortical necrosis of cattle and sheep. Fits in general will be controlled especially those ushered in by symptoms of fear and which tend to return at irregular intervals. There is a general absence of pain.

Strophanthus

Kombe Seed. *N.O.* Apolynaceae. The Ø is prepared from seeds dissolved in alcohol.

Strophanthus produces an increase in the contractile power of striped muscle. It acts especially on the heart increasing systole.

Renal System. There is an increase in the amount of urine passed. Albuminuria may be present.

Female Genital System. Bleeding from uterus.

Respiratory System. Difficult breathing due to lung congestion. Oedema of lungs sometimes arises.

Cardiac System. Heart's action weak with irregular pulse.

Skin. Severe urticaria. Oedema of subcutaneous tissues.

Extremities. Legs become oedematous and swollen. Dropsical conditions in general.

USES

This is a useful remedy to help remove oedema and to tone up heart muscle. It is a safe and useful diuretic especially for the older animal.

Strychninum

Alkaloid of Nux Vomica.   The Ø is prepared from trituration with lactose.

This alkaloid stimulates the motor centres of the spinal cord and increases the depth of respiration. All reflexes are rendered more active.

Eyes.   Dilated pupils. Spasmodic contraction of ocular muscles. Twitching of eyelids.

Alimentary System.   Swallowing is difficult. In the dog and cat vomiting occurs. Bowels are inactive.

Respiratory System.   Very difficult breathing. Spasm of laryngeal muscles.

Extremities.   Rigidity of neck muscles. Stiffness of back with jerking and twitching of limbs and trembling of muscles. Tetanic convulsions set in rapidly.

USES

This remedy may be of use in the early stages of tetanus and similar conditions causing muscular contractions. Post-distemper chorea has also been helped.

Sulfonal

Derivative of Coal Tar.   The Ø is prepared from solution in alcohol or trituration with lactose.

This substance affects the central nervous system causing irregular gait and twitchings with incoordination of muscles.

Renal System.   Scanty reddish urine with albuminuria. Increased desire.

Respiratory System.   Difficult breathing due to lung congestion.

Extremities.   Staggering movements. Stiffenss with paralytic tendency.

Skin.   Purpura with dark red appearance.

USES

This is one of the remedies which may be of use in cerebro-cortical necrosis in cattle and sheep. It may also be of value in post-distempter paraplegia and chorea.

Sulphur

The Element.   The Ø is prepared from solution in alcohol or trituration of sulphur flowers.

Sulphur has a wide ranging action, chief among objective symptoms being a skin rash which is aggravated by heat. Body orifices become red.

Eyes.   Ulceration of eyelids with keratitis. Ophthalmia tends to become chronic.

Ears.   Chronic discharges.

Alimentary System.   There is moderate thirst with redness and swelling of throat.

Renal System.   Increased urination. The urine may be purulent.

Respiratory System.   Rattling of mucus in the lungs. There is a tendency to pleuritic affections.

Skin.   Redness and itching, worse from heat. Wounds may suppurate easily.

USES

This is a useful remedy in eczema rubrum of dogs and cats. Skin conditions tend to be foul-smelling and musty. Abdominal conditions associated with portal stasis and tympany should benefit. Sulphur has the property of aiding the action of other remedies, and is often used in this connection as an inter-current remedy.

Sulphur Iodatum

Sulphur Iodide.   The Ø is prepared from trituration of the salt with lactose.

This salt produces mainly skin symptoms such as papular eruptions with a tendency to pustules and boils. Itching and erythema is common with eczema of a purulent nature.

USES

It should be considered in obstinate skin affections where redness and itching are long-standing and possibly being dependent on constitutional illness.

Sulphuricum Acidum

Sulphuric Acid.   The Ø is prepared from dilution in distilled water.

This acid produces a tendency to gangrene of wounds after mechanical injury.

Eyes. Intra-ocular haemorrhages following injury. Redness of conjunctiva.

Alimentary System. Gums bleed easily.

Skin. Small haemorrhages producing a livid bruised look. Haemorrhages from orifices, the blood being dark. Carbuncles and boils supervene after injuries.

USES

It may be of value in haemorrhagic skin conditions like purpura. In cases of mechanical injury when wounds do not heal easily.

Symphtyum

Comfrey. *N.O.* Boraginaceae. The Ø is prepared from whole fresh plant and root.

The root of this plant produces a substance which stimulates growth of epithelium on ulcerated surfaces, and hastens union of bone in fractures.

USES

This remedy should always be given as a routine in fracture treatment as an aid to healing. Together with other vulneraries like Arnica it is indicated in the treatment of injuries generally. It is also a prominent eye remedy.

Syzygium

Jumbul. *N.O.* Myrtaceae. The Ø is prepared from trituration of seeds and subsequent dilution in alcohol.

This plant exerts an action on the pancreas and this determines its chief use in practice.

USES

In diabetes where it reduces the specific gravity of the urine and reduces thirst and controls urine output.

Tarentula Cubensis

Cuban Spider.   The Ø is prepared from trituration of whole insect.

The poison of the Cuban spider produces a toxic condition with septic complications.

Renal System.   Difficulty in passing urine which may contain blood.

Skin.   Papular reddish eruption. Carbuncles and boils develop. The skin assumes a purplish appearance. Abscesses which appear are very painful.

USES

This is a useful remedy in septic conditions which tend to produce a purplish colour of the skin. The lymphatic system may be involved and the remedy is likely to be of value in lymphangitis especially with septic complications. Abscesses may benefit if they are acute and attended by pain.

Tarentula Hispanica

Spanish Spider.   The Ø is prepared from trituration of whole insect.

Hysterical states are occasioned by this poison. There is a stimulatory effect on the uro-genital system.

Head.   Shaking due to tendency to hysteria.

USES

This remedy should be of value in canine hysteria especially if associated with genital excitement. It could be useful in satyriasis. Also in treating animals exhibiting uncertain temper.

Tellurium

The Metal.   The Ø is prepared from trituration with lactose.

This element exerts an influence on skin, eyes and ears. There is also an action on the sacral region.

Eyes.   The lids become thickened. There is generalised inflammation. Cataract may develop. Conjunctivitis may be pustular.

Ears.   Eczema behind ears. Inflammation of inner and outer ears.

Extremities.   Sacral region becomes sensitive to touch.

Skin.   Herpetic eruptions. Lesions on skin tend to assume an annular form.

USES

Certain forms of ear canker will benefit and it has been used frequently in this connection. Ringworm has also responded especially when lesions are circular in shape and distributed evenly on both sides of the body. It has a long action in the system and should not be repeated too frequently.

Terebinthinae

Turpentine.   The Ø is prepared from solution in rectified spirit.

Haemorrhages are produced from mucous surfaces. Urinary symptoms are prominent.

Alimentary System.   The tongue is red, dry and swollen. Abdomen becomes distended. Gastro-enteritis with dysentery.

Renal System.   Difficulty in urination. Acute nephritis with bloody urine. Cystitis causing increase in attempts to pass urine.

Female Genital System.   Bleeding from uterus, especially after parturition. Uterine inflammation may extend to the peritoneum.

Respiratory System.   Difficulty in breathing. Bleeding from lungs.

Cardiac System.   Small weak pulse.

Skin.   Erythamatous papular eruption. Urticaria. Dropsical states with small haemorrhages.

USES

This is a prominent remedy in acute nephritis associated with haematuria and when the urine smells of turpentine or sweetish this odour had been likened to that of violets. The nephritis may be associated with cystitis and here again blood-stained urine will be present. It also has a use in the treatment of gaseous bloat in ruminants. Some forms of puerperal fever will be influenced especially when accompanied by kidney inflammation producing the characteristic urine odour.

Teucrium Marum

Cat Thyme.   *N.O.* Labiatae.   The Ø is prepared from the whole fresh plant.

This plant has an action on both the respiratory and alimentary systems.

Eyes.   Red and inflamed. Conjunctivitis.

Respiratory System.   Nasal obstruction. Frequent sneezing. Dry cough.

Alimentary System.   Mucus in mouth. Pharyngitis. Increased appetite. Tympany with colic. Severe diarrhoea. Expels round worms.

Renal System.   Polyuria. Urine of low specific gravity.

USES

This is a useful remedy in some forms of cat influenza showing the typical nasal discharges. It should be remembered also for its ability to expel round worms.

Thlaspi Bursa

Shepherd's Purse.   *N.O.* Cruciferae.   The Ø is prepared from fresh flowering plant.

This plant produces haemorrhages and a uric acid diathesis.

Respiratory System.   Passive bleeding from nose.

Female Genital System.   Uterine haemorrhage. It favours expulsion of blood-clots from the uterus.

Renal System.   Frequency of urination. The urine is turbid and heavy with reddish sediment. Blood-stained urine with cystitis.

USES

Its sphere of action determines its use mainly in affections of the uro-genital system, e.g. acute cystitis and urethritis with the presence of calculi. It may prevent the use of the catheter by its ability to dissolve sandy deposits and small calculi.

Thuja Occidentalis

Arbor Vitae.   *N.O.* Coniferae.   The Ø is prepared from fresh green twigs.

Thuja produces a condition which favours the formation of warty growths and tumours. It acts mainly on the skin and uro-genital system.

Eyes.   Tarsal tumours and warts develop. Eyelids become agglutinated.

Male Genital System.   Balanitis and prostatitis.

Skin.   Warts and herpetic eruptions are commonly seen. The scrotum and sheath are particularly affected in the horse, while in cattle, the neck and abdomen are favourite sites.

USES

This remedy is of great value in the treatment of skin conditions accompanied by the presence of warty growths which tend to bleed easily. Papillomatous warts will be especially influenced, and should respond to treatment when they are internal, e.g. in the bladder, as well as external.

Thyroidinum

Thyroid Gland.   The Ø is prepared from trituration with lactose or solution in distilled water.

Anaemia, emaciation and muscular weakness are associated with excess of thyroid secretion.

Eyes.   Dilation and protrusion of eyes and pupils.

Cardiac System.   The heart rate is increased.

USES

This remedy is of value in alopecia and allied skin conditions, e.g. dry eczema. It influences also the growth of mammary tumours in the bitch. Some forms of jaundice are helped. Conditions accompanied by acceleration of heart's action should benefit if other remedies fail to act.

Trifolium Pratense

Red Clover.   *N.O.* Leguminosae.   The Ø is prepared from flower heads.

Produces marked salivation with swelling of salivary glands.

Alimentary System.   Salivation. The throat becoms swollen causing difficulty in swallowing.

Respiratory System.   Paroxysmal cough accompanied by thin mucous secretion.

USES

Affections of the mouth such as stomatitis leading to salivation may benefit, especially when accompanied by swelling of sub-maxillary glands.

Trillium Pendulum

White Beth-Root.   *N.O.* Liliaceae.   The Ø is prepared from fresh root.

Haemorrhages are produced along with blood-stained mucous diarrhoea.

Alimentary System.   Bleeding from gums, also from stomach. Chronic diarrhoea leading to dysentery.

Female Genital System.   Bleeding from uterus, blood bright red. Tendency to prolapse.

Respiratory System.   Bleeding from lungs with coughing.

USES

This remedy has some value in threatened abortion preceded by blood-stained discharge. Specific conditions which may be helped are mucosal disease of calves and dysentery of swine. In small animal practice dogs presented with symptoms of warfarin poisoning may respond to treatment if this is carried out promptly. Such cases should be selected according to the nature and location of the haemorrhage.

Triticum

Couch Grass.   *N.O.* Graminae.   The Ø is prepared from fresh plant.

This grass acts on the bladder and uro-genital system causing difficult urination.

Renal System.   Frequent urging to urinate. Gravelly deposits in the urine. Pyelitis and cystitis develop. The prostate gland may become enlarged.

USES

This remedy will be found to alleviate certain types of cystitis and kidney disease. Its action on the prostate gland should not be overlooked.

Uranium Nitricum

Uranium Nitrate.   The Ø is prepared from solution in distilled water.

Glycosuria and polyuria are the main objective symptoms associated with the provings of this salt.

Eyes.   The eyelids become agglutinated.

Alimentary System.   Thirst is a prominent symptom. In the dog and cat vomiting is frequent especially after drinking. Abdominal discomfort is evidenced by flatulence and there may be ascites, due to liver degeneration.

Renal System.   Great amounts of urine are passed of an acid reaction. There is a diabetic tendency.

USES

This is a valuable remedy in diabetic states in the dog and in similar conditions characterised by emaciation and polyuria. Its beneficial action on the liver aids the dispersal of abdominal fluid and reduces or eliminates the tendency to vomition.

Urea

The Ø is prepared from solution in distilled water or trituration of dried substance.

This substance brings about a condition associated with enlargement of various glands. It causes dropsy due to renal malfunction. The liver and eyes may also be affected.

Eyes.   Itching with excessive lachrymation.

Alimentary System.   Enlargement of liver. Severe ascites.

Renal System.   Urging to urinate pronounced. Urine contains heavy sediment. Polyuria associated with dropsy.

USES

This remedy should be considered in threatened uraemia, especially when associated with dropsical states. Also in generalised nephritic and cystitic conditions accompanied by albuminuria.

Urtica Urens

Stinging Nettle. *N.O.* Urticaceae. The Ø is prepared from fresh plant in flower.

The nettle causes agalactia with a tendency to the formation of calculi. There is a general uric acid diathesis with urticarial swellings also present.

Alimentary System. Mucous ulceration of the large gut leading to chronic diarrhoea.

Female Genital System. Diminished secretion of milk. Bleeding from uterus. Enlargement of mammary glands with oedema of tissue.

Skin. Itching erythematous eruptions, urticaria and oedematous plaques.

Renal System. Acute nephritis. Uric acid deposits in urine.

USES

An extremely useful remedy in various renal and other conditions. In prevention of calculi it acts by thickening the urine which thus contains increased deposits of urates and other salts. It helps restore normal milk flow and is therefore suitable for use in cases of agalactia, particularly in the sow where this condition is of frequent occurrence, and in first-calving heifers which show oedema of udder. Nephritis associated with skin lesions may call for its use. These lesions are frequently oedematous. It helps promote normal urination and has been used successfully in many cases of suppression.

Ustillago Maydis

Corn Smut. *N.O.* Fungi. The Ø is prepared from trituration of fungus with lactose.

This substance has an affinity for the genital organs of both male and female, particularly the latter where the uterus is markedly affected.

Skin. Alopecia of various parts. Eczema with rough dry hair.

Female Genital System. Discharge of blood from uterus, blood being bright red and partly clotted. Hypertrophied flabby condition of uterine muscle. Post-partum haemorrhage. Tendency to prolapse. Early abortion in the pregnant animal.

Male Genital System. Relaxed organs with swelling of testicles. In dogs excessive desire is a prominent symptom.

USES

Various forms of uterine discharges from muco-purulent to haemorrhagic come within its sphere of action. It could have a place in the treatment of animals which have a tendency to abortion and in the control of accompanying haemorrhage. In the male dog it has given good results in controlling masturbation and in this connection should be tried before castration is undertaken as an alternative.

Uva Ursi

Bear Berry.   *N.O.* Eucaceae.   The Ø is prepared from fresh leaves.

The active principles are associated with disturbances of the urinary system, particularly cystitis.

Renal System.   Difficult urination with bladder inflammation and tenesmus. Urine may contain blood, pus and mucus. Kidney involvement is usually confined to the pelvis causing a purulent inflammation.

Female Genital System.   There may be bleeding from the uterus.

USES

One of the main remedies in the treatment of cystitis and other conditions where pus in the urine is of more or less constant occurrence.

Valeriana

Valerian. *N.O.* Valerianaceae. The Ø is prepared from fresh root.

Affections of the nervous system are associated with this plant, hysteria being a prominent symptom.

Nervous System. Hysterical fits. Hypersensitivity to stimuli.

Alimentary System. Flatulence. Aversion to food. Bloated abdomen.

Extremities. Jerking and trembling of lower limbs particularly.

USES

A useful remedy in controlling hysteria in the dog.

Vanadium

The Metal. The Ø is prepared from trituration with lactose.

This metal aids the oxygen-carrying power of the blood.

USES

It is of use in marasmic conditions and wasting diseases. It aids the production of leucocytes, phagocytes in particular, and is therefore of use in combating bacterial toxins. Degenerative conditions of the vascular system are helped.

Veratrum Album

White Hellebore. *N.O.* Liliaceae. The Ø is prepared from fresh roots.

A picture of collapse is presented by the action of this plant, with cold extremities and cyanosis.

Eyes. Increased secretions. Heavy appearance of lids.

Alimentary System. Increased appetite. Purging and vomiting, watery diarrhoea with exhaustion.

Respiratory System.   Rattling of mucus. Cough from lung congestion.

Cardiac System.   Rapid weak pulse.

Extremities.   Tenderness over joints.

Skin.   Extreme coldness.

USES

A useful remedy in gastro-enteritis with threatened collapse, e.g. in coli-bacillosis of calves. It is a useful cardiac stimulant in cases of collapse. It is sometimes combined with Arsenic Alb. and China in the treatment of diarrhoea where it is useful in controlling dehydration. In the horse it may be useful in cases of flatulent colic. This remedy should be considered in any condition where the body becomes very cold when associated with collapse and diarrhoea.

Veratrum Viridum

Green Hellebore.   *N.O.* Liliaceae.   The Ø is prepared from fresh roots.

This plant causes a fall in both systolic and diastolic blood-pressure.

Eyes.   Redness with dilated pupils.

Alimentary System.   In the dog and cat there may be vomiting immediately after eating.

Respiratory System. Congestion of lungs with difficult breathing.

Renal System.   Scanty cloudy urine.

Female Genital System.   Rigidity of os uteri.

Cardiac System.   Auricular fibrillation. Pulse soft, slow and weak.

Extremities.   Twitching of limbs. Pain and tenderness over joints.

Skin.   Erythematous itching, especially associated with symptoms of nervous disturbance.

USES

Of use in septic feverish states showing alternation of temperature. General congestive states should benefit. It could be of benefit in ringwomb in ewes, and also in pulmonary congestion with threatened oedema.

Vespa

Wasp Venom.   The Ø is prepared from the fresh insect.

This poison is associated with skin symptoms and also with affections of the female genital system.

Head.   Swollen and oedematous. Erysipelatous inflammation of eyelids. Conjunctivae become injected. Swelling of mouth and throat.

Renal System.   Increased urination. Urine may be high-coloured.

Female Genital System.   Affections of ovaries. Acrid discharge from os uteri.

Skin.   Erythema with severe itching and burning. Oedematous swellings.

USES

Affections of the ovary may benefit, especially acute inflammation. Its action on the skin may determine its choice.

Viburnum Opulis

Cranberry.   *N.O.* Capufoliaceae.   The Ø is prepared from fresh bark.

Muscular cramps are associated with the action of this plant. The female genital system is also affected.

Alimentary System.   Lack of appetite. Colicky pains are evident with sensitivity over the umbilicus.

Female Genital System.   The uterus is principally affected producing a tendency to abortion in the first quarter of pregnancy. Sterility is a common sequel.

Renal System.   Frequent urging to urinate, the urine being pale and copious.

Extremities.   Stiffness and weakness of lower limbs.

USES

Principally used for the treatment of animals with a history of repeated miscarriages, mainly in small animal practice. The Ø has been successfully used to produce abortion in unwanted pregnancies.

Vinca Minor

Lesser Periwinkle.   *N.O.* Apocynaceae.   The Ø is prepared from whole fresh plant.

The skin is affected, eczema-like symptoms being a common feature. Haemorrhages from various parts also occur.

Alimentary System.   Difficult swallowing due to ulceration of throat.

Female Genital System.   Bleeding from uterus.

Skin. Itching eczema. Redness and pain after scratching. Pustular eruptions.

USES

Of use as an anti-allergic skin remedy when erythema and itching arise. The action on the throat should be noted and also the tendency to haemorrhage which may determine its use in skin conditions.

Vipera

Poison of the Viper. The Ø is prepared from dilution of venom in alcohol.

This poison causes paresis of the lower limbs with a tendency to paraplegia. Symptoms extend upwards.

Face and Head. Skin and subcutaneous tissues become excessively swollen with livid tongue and swollen lips.

Alimentary System. Enlargement of liver. Disturbance of liver function produces jaundice.

Extremities. Acute inflammation of veins of lower limbs. Oedema of dependent structures.

Skin. Boils, pimples and carbuncles may develop.

USES

Venous congestion producing oedema and swelling come within its sphere of action. It could prove useful in the treatment of septic lymphangitis. Liver disease with accompanying jaundice may benefit in the acute stage.

Yohimbinum

N.O. Rubiaceae. The Ø is prepared from solution of alkaloid in alcohol or trituration of dried substance.

This substance acts mainly on the sexual organs and the central nervous system.

Alimentary System. Copious salivation is the main symptom.

Sexual Sphere. Its action is mainly seen in the male producing satyriasis, often accompanied by symptoms of urethral inflammation such as mucous discharge.

USES

Should be considered as one of the remedies which could prove of benefit when treating hyper-sexuality in the male dog.

Zincum Metallicum

Zinc. The Ø is prepared from trituration with lactose.

This element produces a state of anaemia where there occurs a decrease in the number of red cells.

Head. There is a tendency to fall towards the left side. Cerebral symptoms predominate.

Eyes. Lachrymation. Heaviness and twitching of eyelids. Conjunctiva becomes red and inflamed.

Ears. Inflammation of inner and outer ears.

Alimentary System. Blisters appear on the tongue. Dryness of mouth with difficult swallowing. In the dog and cat vomiting occurs. Tympany of abdomen with tenderness over umbilicus. Enlargement of liver with signs of flatulent colic.

Extremities. Lameness and weakness with trembling and twitching of muscles.

USES

This is a useful remedy in suppressed feverish conditions and septic states of long-standing. It may have a place in the treatment of anaemia. Recurrent cases of flatulent colic in the horse should benefit and also cerebro-cortical necrosis.

Zingiber

Ginger. *N.O.* Zingiberaceae. The Ø is prepared from dried rhizome.

The powdered root produces a state of debility of the digestive tract. There is also a lesser action on the respiratory and uro-genital systems.

Alimentary System. Rumbling of flatus. Increased thirst. Diarrhoea with signs of colic.

Renal System. Frequent urination. Urine thick and turbid.

Respiratory System. Dry cough with difficult breathing.

USES

Digestive upsets with colicky symptoms should benefit, e.g. flatulent colic in the horse.

Materia Medica of the Nosodes, and Oral Vaccines

A nosode is a disease product obtained from any affected part of the system in a case of illness and thereafter potentised, e.g. Fowl Pest nosode from the respiratory secretions of affected birds. In specific, i.e. bacterial, viral or protozoal disease, the causative organism may or may not be present in the material, and the efficacy of the nosode in no way depends on the organism being present. The response of the tissue to invasion by bacteria or viruses results in the formation of substances which are in effect the basis of the nosode.

An oral vaccine is prepared from the actual organism which causes disease and may derive from filtrates containing only the exotoxins of the bacteria, or from emulsions containing both bacteria and their toxins. These filtrates and emulsions are then potentised and become oral vaccines. Nowadays it is the custom to use the two terms synonymously.

There are two different ways of employing nosodes: viz. 1. therapeutically and 2. prophylactically.

When we employ nosodes for treatment we may use them in the condition from which the nosode was derived, e.g. Distemperinum in the treatment of distemper. This method may be termed isopathic, i.e. treatment with a substance taken from an animal suffering from the *same* disease, or we may employ the nosode in any condition the symptoms of which resemble the symptom-complex of the particular nosode, e.g. the use of Psorinum in the treatment of the special kind of eczema which appears in the provings of that nosode. This method may be termed homoeopathic, i.e. treatment with a substance taken from an animal suffering from a *similar* disease. In this connection it must be remembered that all the great nosodes have been proved in their own right, i.e. each has its own particular drug picture. Many veterinary nosodes have been developed in recent years but no provings exist for them and they are used almost solely in the treatment or prevention of the associated diseases.

Autonosodes.   This particular type of nosode is prepared from material provided by the patient alone, e.g. pus from a chronic sinus or fistula and after potentisation used for the treatment of the same patient. Many examples of this could be quoted but I think it is sufficient to explain the theory. Autonosodes are usually employed in refractory cases where well indicated remedies have failed to produce the desired response and frequently they produce striking results.

Oral Vaccines.   As with nosodes, oral vaccines may be used both therapeutically and prophylactically. If the condition is caused wholly by bacterial or viral invasion the use of the oral vaccine is frequently attended by spectacular success but this is less likely when there is an underlying chronic condition complicating an acute infection. Here we may need the help of constitutional and other remedies.

Bowel Nosodes.   The bowel nosodes are usually included under the heading of oral vaccines as the potentised vaccines are prepared from cultures of the organisms themselves. As a preliminary introduction to the study of the bowel nosodes let us consider the role of the E. coli organism. In the normal healthy animal the function of the E. coli bacteria is beneficial rendering complex materials resulting from the digestive process into simpler substances. If, however, the patient is subjected to any change, e.g. stress, which affects the intestinal mucosa, the balance between normal health and illness will be upset and the E. coli organisms may then be said to have become pathogenic. This change in the patient need not be a detrimental one, as the administration of potentised homoeopathic remedies can bring it about. The illness therefore may originate in the patient which causes the bacteria to change their behaviour.

   In laboratory tests it has been noticed that from a patient who had previously yielded only E. coli there suddenly appeared a large percentage of non-lactose fermenting bacilli of a type associated with the pathogenic group of typhoid and paratyphoid disease. Since the non-lactose fermenting bacilli had appeared after a latent period of 10–14 days following the administration of the remedy it would seem that the homoepathic potentised remedy had changed the bowel flora. The pathogenic germ in this case was the result of vital stimulation set up in the patient by the potentised remedy; the germ was not the *cause* of any change. Each germ or bacillus is associated with its own peculiar symptom-picture and certain conclusions may be made from clinical and laboratory observation. These may be summarised as follows:

a) The specific organism is related to the disease.
b) The specific organism is related to the homoeopathic remedy.
c) The homoeopathic remedy is related to the disease.

The bowel nosodes which concern us in veterinary practice are as follows: 1. Morgan-Bach; 2. Proteus-Bach; 3. Gaertner-Bach; 4. Dys Co-Bach; 5. Sycotic Co-Paterson.

Morgan-Bach. Clinical observations have revealed the symptom-picture of the bacillus Morgan to cover in general digestive and respiratory systems with an action also on fibrous tissues and skin. It is used mainly in eczema of young dogs combined with an appropriate remedy, compatible ones being Sulphur, Graphites, Petroleum and Psorinium.

Proteus-Bach. The central and peripheral nervous systems figure prominently in the provings of this nosode, e.g. convulsions and seizures together with spasm of the peripheral circulation: cramping of muscles is a common feature: angio-neurotic oedema frequently occurs and there is marked sensitivity to ultra-violet light. Associated remedies are Cuprum Metallicum, and Natrium Muriaticum.

Gaertner-Bach. Marked emaciation or malnutrition is associated with this nosode. Chronic gastro-enteritis occurs and there is a tendency for the animal to become infested with worms. There is an inability to digest fat. Associated remedies are Mercurius, Phosphorus and Silicea.

Dys Co-Bach. This nosode is chiefly concerned with the digestive and cardiac systems.

Pyloric spasm occurs with retention of digested stomach contents leading to vomiting. There is functional disturbance of the heart's action, sometimes seen in nervous dogs, usually associated with tension.

Associated remedies are Arsenicum Album, Argentum Nitricum and Kalmia Latifolia.

Sycotic Co-Paterson. The keynote of this nosode is sub-acute or chronic inflammation of mucous membranes especially those of the intestinal tract where a chronic catarrhal enteritis occurs. Chronic bronchitis and nasal catarrh are met with.

Associated remedies are Mercurius Corrosivus, Nitricum Acidum and Hydrastis.

Main Indications for the use of the Bowel Nosodes

When a case is presented showing one or two leading symptoms which suggest a particular remedy we should employ that remedy, if necessary in varying potencies before abandoning it and resorting to another if unsatisfactory results ensue. In chronic disease there may be conflicting symptoms which suggest several competing remedies and it is here that the bowel nosodes may be used with advantage. A study of the associated remedies will usually lead us to the particular nosode to be employed. The question of potency and repetition of dosage assumes special importance when considering the use of bowel nosodes. The mental and emotional symptoms which are frequently present in illness in the human being are not available to a veterinary surgeon and he therefore concerns himself with objective signs and pathological change. The low to medium potencies, e.g. 6c. – 30c. are more suitable for this purpose than the higher ones and can be safely administered daily for a few days. Bowel nosodes are deep-acting remedies and should not be repeated until a few months have elapsed since the first prescription.

Main Guide to the Use of Nosodes

1. Therapeutic Use. Usually the 30c potency is used but in the treatment of some acute conditions it may be necessary to employ the higher ones. In many cases the nosode can be used by itself, e.g. Variolinum in cow pox or E. coli in white scour, where a dose of the nosode three times per day for two days is given and if necessary repeated every second day for three doses. Most of them, however, are combined with selected remedies in the treatment of various conditions either associated with the specific disease or in those which provide a symptom-picture resembling the provings of the particular nosode in question, e.g. the use of Psorinum in eczema.

2. Prophylactic Use. When we use any nosode for the prevention of disease we employ it in 30c potency. There are different approaches to this problem but the one favoured by the author is as follows:

One dose is given night and morning for three days followed by one per month for six months. This provides a good level of protection after the first week which is subsequently re-inforced over the next few months. One of the benefits of oral vaccination, apart from its safety and absence of side-effects, is that protection can be provided at an early age, e.g. a puppy which is presented for vaccination against distemper and/or Parvovirus disease can be protected at 3–4 weeks of age instead of having to wait for nine weeks, as is the case when conventional injections are given.

There is some doubt as to how protection by a nosode or oral vaccine is produced. The antibody theory as far as we know appears not to be relevant, but protection seems to be given by rendering the animal less resistance to infection by raising the opsonic index to infection. In other words the entire defence system is stimulated.

The following nosodes are all useful in veterinary practice, either as remedies in their own right, i.e. those which have had provings done on them, or as disease products used in conjunction with indicated remedies in the treatment of conditions from which they were obtained. Those which have their own drug picture include the following.

1. Ambra Grisea.   The Ø is prepared from the tissues of the Sperm
Whale by trituration and subsequent dilution in alcohol.

This substance exerts an influence on the central nervous system
producing hysterical states with a tendency to convulsions. There is also
an action on the digestive and renal systems where colic and polyuria
may occur. The urine may be tinged with blood. A dry burning eczema
may be present. This nosode is chiefly to be thought of in connection
with nervous and urinary conditions, e.g. hysteria and diabetes
insipidus in the dog.

2. Anthracinum.   The Ø is prepared from affected tissue and dissolved in alcohol. This nosode is indicated in the treatment of eruptive
skin diseases which are characterised by boil-like swellings. Cellular
tissue becomes indurated and swelling of associated lymph glands takes
place. The characteristic lesion assumes the form of a hard swelling
with a necrotic centre and surrounded by a blackened rim. Lesions tend
to become gangrenous. Has proved useful in the treatment of adder
bite.

3. Bacillinum.   This is one of the nosodes of tuberculosis and the Ø
is prepared from sputum, triturated and dissolved in alcohol. In veterinary practice its use is confined mainly to the treatment of ringworm in
various species, especially cattle where it has given consistently good
results. It could have a place in the treatment of eczema in general,
combined with indicated remedies.

4. Carcinosin.   This is one of the cancer nosodes, the Ø being prepared from diseased epithelial tissue. It is used in veterinary practice as
an aid in the treatment of mammary tumours in the bitch and other
forms of malignancy involving epithelial tissue. It also has a reputation
as a vermifuge against threadworms but as far as the author knows there
are no records of its use in this connection in the veterinary field. It
could also be of use in some forms of lymphadenitis.

5. Cholesterinum.   The Ø is prepared by trituration and sub
sequent dilution of the natural substance obtained from bile. This
nosode is used in conditions affecting mainly the liver when the func
tion of this gland becomes sluggish and there is a tendency to the pro
duction of gravel and jaundice. It combines well with remedies such a
Lycopodium and Berberis Vulgaris.

6. Corticotrophin (A.C.T.H.).   The Ø is prepared from th
anterior lobe of the pituitary gland by trituration and subsequent dilu
tion in alcohol. It could prove of use in the treatment of digestive an
genito-urinary conditions, e.g. stomatitis, hepatitis and dysentery. Dia

betes insipidus in the dog has responded well to treatment by this substance.

7. Cortisone. This is the hormone prepared by the cortex of the adrenal gland and the Ø is made from the natural substance or from synthetic material, triturated and dissolved in alcohol. The over-prescribing of the crude drug produces a variety of symptoms, those which are of interest to the veterinarian being confined mainly to the skin, where redness, excessive scratching, pigmentation and loss of hair predominate. There is also retention of water in the tissues. The total symptom-picture suggests an artificial Cushing's Disease syndrome. In homoeopathic potency this hormone is of use in the treatment of skin diseases using various potencies and should always be considered as an antidote to the excessive use of the crude drug.

8. D.N.A. The Ø is prepared from the natural substance, dissolved in alcohol. The provings of this material have produced a variety of symptoms based mainly on the digestive and locomotor systems and the skin. It could prove of value in the treatment of eczema and pancreatitis in the dog and also in some forms of arthritis resistant to other remedies.

9. Epihysterinum. The source of the Ø is blood from a uterine fibroid, and after trituration dissolved in alcohol. It has a reputation as a useful remedy in controlling uterine haemorrhage from whatever source and could profitably be combined with selected remedies in this connection.

10. Folliculinum. This is one of the ovarian hormones, the Ø being prepared from a solution in alcohol. In veterinary practice it has proved of great value in the treatment of miliary eczema in the cat and hormonal alopecia in the bitch. It combines well with selected remedies such as Lycopodium, Natrum Muriaticum and Selenium.

11. Hippomanes. This substance is prepared from allantois fluid, the Ø being made from dilutions in alcohol. It is one of the lesser used remedies but it could prove useful in the treatment of enlarged prostate in the older dog and also in radial paralysis.

12. Hippozaeninum. This nosode has been in existence a long time having been made from Glanders, a notifiable equine disease no longer encountered in the British Isles. The Ø is prepared from trituration of diseased material and thereafter dissolved in alcohol. It has a wide range of use in many catarrhal conditions which are characterised by glairy or glutinous discharges, e.g. sinusitis, ozaena and ulceration of nasal cartilages. It has been used effectively in the treatment of post-influenzal bronchitis.

13. Hirudin.   This substance is obtained from the common leech, the Ø being prepared from trituration of the head and subsequent dilution in Thymol. The action is related to that of snake venoms in that there is a tendency for bleeding to take place from orifices. The neck glands become swollen and the heart's action becomes irregular. This remedy could take its place alongside those other related ones, e.g. Crotalus Horridus, Lachesis and Naja Tripudians.

14. Histaminum.   This naturally occurring substance causes dilation of capillary blood-vessels and constricts the bronchi. Gastric and pancreatic secretions are stimulated. The Ø is prepared from the hydrochloride salt. It has a limited use in veterinary practice in conditions relating to the digestive and urinary tracts, viz. colitis and urinary suppression, and also in allergic skin conditions, e.g. urticaria.

15. Hydrophobinum (Lyssin).   This is the nosode of rabies, the Ø being prepared from saliva from a rabid animal, with subsequent dilution in alcohol. In veterinary practice it is a useful remedy in the treatment of those animals showing fear, either of objects or other animals and people. Bright objects may bring on convulsions in susceptible animals. Extreme cases may show excessive salivation and aggressive behaviour.

16. Hypophysis.   The posterior lobe of the pituitary gland is the source of this hormone, the Ø being prepared by maceration in alcohol. It contains an anti-diuretic factor which regulates the activity of the kidney tubules. There is also an action on the smooth muscle of the uterus causing contraction. In veterinary practice it has a use as an auxillary remedy in nephritis and incontinence.

17. Hypothalamus.   The Ø is obtained from the hypothalamus itself, macerated and dissolved in alcohol. Although no actual proving exists for this remedy its use is based on clinical experience. It has a limited use in veterinary practice but could be useful in alopecia and skin complaints in general.

18. Influenzinum.   The nosode of influenza is prepared from respiratory secretions containing the virus and other infective agents and thereafter dissolved in alcohol. It has given good results either as a remedy in its own right in the treatment of influenza and catarrhal conditions of the respiratory tract or combined with indicated remedies. For the oral vaccination of horses it is combined with human influenza strains.

19. Lac caninum.   The Ø is prepared from the milk of the bitch.

This remedy has been used successfully in many cases of septic pharyngitis and tonsillitis together with nasal discharges of various forms. Associated lymph glands become swollen. For a fuller description see the main text.

20. Malandrinum. This nosode has been developed from the condition called Grease in the horse after trituration of affected material. It is used mainly in the treatment of inveterate skin eruptions and discharges and has given good results in cases of Mud Fever. It has a bearing on the treatment of some forms of cow pox and is worth using as a preventive measure against summer mastitis in cattle.

21. Medorrhinum. The Ø is prepared from gonorrhoeal discharges after dilution in alcohol. This nosode has a limited use in veterinary practice but it has been used in various joint affections together with some forms of eczema. It may also have a beneficial effect in cases of ear canker and chronic nasal discharges.

22. Morbillinum. The nosode of measles, prepared from infected material has also a limited use in veterinary practice, but it has proved beneficial in the treatment of eczema in dogs when the condition takes the form of multiple round measles-like eruptions, particularly on the abdomen. Catarrhal conditions affecting the ears and respiratory organs may also benefit.

23. Oopherinum. This is another of the ovarian hormones prepared from ovarian extract, and after trituration, dissolved in alcohol. Its main use in veterinary practice is in the treatment of miliary eczema and could be alternated with other nosodes such as Folliculinum and Orchitinum. It could also influence the tendency to obesity which frequently follows ovaro-hysterectomy in the bitch.

24. Orchitinum. This nosode is prepared from testicular extract after trituration. Like the previous remedy it is used principally in the treatment of miliary eczema in the neutered animal especially the male. It should be combined with remedies such as Lycopodium and Thallium Acetas.

25. Osteo-Arthritic Nosode. The Ø is prepared from fluid taken from an osteoarthritic joint, and dissolved in alcohol. It is a remedy which has a place in the treatment of degenerative joint conditions especially in the older dog. Ringbone in the horse and also spavin may also benefit. It may be used on its own or combined with other remedies.

26. Pancreatinum.   The Ø is prepared from pancreatic extract after trituration, It is used in various disorders of the pancreas either on its own or combined with selected remedies to suit the individual case. In pancreatitis it may be used along with Trypsinum.

27. Parathyroidinum. (Parathormone)   The Ø is prepared from the parathyroid hormone after extraction and solution in alcohol. This hormone regulates calcium metabolism and calcium may be increased or decreased in blood and urine. Phosphaturia also occurs. Excess secretion causes bone weakness with possible fracture and deformity. The digestive system is also affected giving rise to loss of appetite and constipation. The muscular system becomes involved, the animal showing weakness and loss of muscle tone. Heart muscle is also affected. In practice it may be used in various conditions affecting the musculoskeletal system particularly, e.g. osteoporosis.

28. Parotidinum.   This is the nosode of mumps and in veterinary practice it is a useful remedy in the treatment of cases of parotitis and associated glandular swellings. It may be used either on its own or combined with indicated remedies. It could prove useful in the treatment of orchitis.

29. Pepsinum.   This nosode is prepared from gastric juices containing the enzyme pepsin. It is used particularly as an aid to digestion in combination with other digestive remedies, e.g. Nux Vomica, to promote appetite.

30. Pertussin.   The nosode of whooping cough has a limited use in veterinary practice but it has proved beneficial in aiding recovery in kennel cough combined with selected remedies. It may prove useful in long-standing bronchitic states.

31. Psorinum.   The Ø is prepared from fluid taken from a scabies vesicle. This nosode has had an extensive proving and is used in veterinary practice in the treatment of intractable skin diseases of a suppressive nature; also in ear canker. One of the guiding symptoms which point to its use is an offensive smell with a desire to seek warmth. The skin is usually dry and the coat harsh when this remedy is indicated. For a fuller description see main text.

32. Pyrogenium.   The Ø in this case is made from decaying protein matter. A thorough proving has also been carried out. It is used in a wide variety of septic and putrid conditions where the main guiding symptom is a discrepancy between pulse and temperature. Conditions where it has done excellent work include puerperal metritis and summer mastitis. For a fuller description see main text.

33. R.N.A. The Ø is prepared from the natural substance. Provings of R.N.A. produced a variety of symptoms, those of interest to the veterinarian being related to the skin, genito-urinary, digestive and circulatory systems. It could prove useful in the treatment of biliary and pancreatic troubles; also in vaginitis and leukaemia combined with related remedies.

34. Scarlatinum. The nosode of scarlet fever. The main use in veterinary practice for this remedy is in the treatment of erythematous skin rashes where it can be combined with other remedies, e.g. Belladonna. Also in pharyngitis and nephritis with one or other of the Mercurius remedies.

35. Staphylococcus. The particular species of staphylococcus used in veterinary practice is S. Aureus. It has a wide range of use when potentised ranging from treatment of skin abscesses and anal gland infection to mastitis in cattle and sheep. It should always be considered along with indicated remedies where staphylococcal infection is thought to be present.

36. Streptococcus. This nosode may either be used as one distinct strain or type or more often as a composite containing different strains of both haemolytic and non-haemolytic varieties. Again the range of use in practice is wide and embraces such common conditions as mastitis in cows and joint-ill in calves. It is frequently used on its own.

37. Thalamus. The source of the Ø for this substance is nerve material taken from the region of the encephalon in the brain. It has a limited use in veterinary practice but it could prove helpful in aiding other remedies in conditions associated with inco-ordination, e.g. cerebro-cortical necrosis in sheep and cattle. It could also be useful in hepatic and pancreatic conditions.

38. Thyreotrophic hormone. The source of this hormone is the anterior lobe of the pituitary gland. It exerts a powerful action on the thyroid gland where oversecretion produces hypertrophy of the gland along with an increase in heart rate. The indications for its use in homoeopathic practice are based on clinical observations, and include such conditions as tachycardia, dyspepsia and arthritis. Some cases of pigmentation of hair may also respond. It also has some reputation as a vermifuge.

39. Thyroidinum.   The Ø is prepared by trituration of fresh thyroid gland and subsequent dilution. This is a useful nosode in veterinary practice and has a wide range of action. Conditions such as alopoecia, deficiency of milk and puerperal fevers all come within its range of action. It should be combined with iodum in the treatment of conditions affecting the thyroid gland itself, e.g. goitre and myxoedema. For fuller description see main text.

40. Trypsinum.   This is one of the pancreatic enzymes and the Ø is prepared from pancreatic extract after trituration. It is used in the treatment of pancreatitis and as an aid to digestion. Clinical cases likely to benefit from its use show bulky undigested stools and less frequently pale semi-formed stools.

41. Tuberculinum aviare.   This is the nosode of avian tuberculosis and is used in veterinary practice as a remedy to aid convalescence after influenza and bronchitis and for protection against tuberculosis in the fowl.

42. Tuberculinum Bovinum.   This nosode, prepared from a bovine source, is used particularly as a prophylactic in bovine mastitis where it should be given every three months on a routine herd basis in alternation with other mastitis nosodes. Apart from this specific action it will have a beneficial effect generally on the herd.

43. Vaccininum.   This nosode is prepared from smallpox vaccine, triturated and dissolved in alcohol. It has a generalised action and may be used in the treatment of conjunctivitis and chronic eczema when lesions tend to coalesce and suppurate.

44. Variolinum.   This is the nosode of smallpox itself and is prepared in the same way as the above from diseased tissue containing the virus. It has been used successfully in practice both for treatment and protection of cow and goat pox. In an outbreak of this disease all in-contact animals should be given a course of this nosode.

In addition to the above nosodes others have been prepared against the following diseases.

1. Brucella Abortus.   This nosode contains both Br. Abortus and Br. Melitensis strains and can be used as a prophylactic measure. It is entirely without risk or prejudice to blood-testing. Protection should start at 9 months of age.

2. Caliciviruses.   This nosode covers the main cat viruses which affect the mouth, naso-pharynx and respiratory systems. It has been prepared from infected secretions.

3. Canine Distemper. This nosode contains virus obtained from infected mesenteric glands and blood. It is usually employed as an aid in the treatment of distemper, in ascending potencies ranging from 30c. to CM. It gives very good results and hastens the action of other remedies.

4. Colibacillosis. This nosode is made from various strains of E. coli and can be obtained either as a single remedy or as a combination of different strains. The most successful one used in the control and treatment of white scour in calves is one based on a human source.

5. Equine Influenza. The nosode used in practice contains all known strains of human and equine virus. Apart from giving good results as a prophylactic measure it can be used to hasten convalescence after influenza and will remove any side-effects which may arise from conventional vaccination.

6. Equid Herpesvirus 1. This nosode is used as a prophylactic measure along with the influenza nosode to give protection to horses at risk. It has proved to be very effective.

7. Feline Infectious Anaemia. Prepared from the blood of an affected animal and used both for treatment and prevention.

8. Feline Infectious Peritonitis. Prepared from infected peritoneal fluid and used as above.

9. Feline Panleucopenia. Prepared from mesenteric lymph glands and blood from an affected animal and used as above.

10. Feline Viral Rhinotracheitis. Prepared from respiratory and nasal discharges. Used as a remedy on its own or with selected remedies for treatment. Has given good results as an oral vaccine.

11. Feline Leukaemia. Prepared from the blood of an affected animal and from a lymphosarcoma tumour. Experience has shown that this nosode has helped in the treatment of some cases of Felv. It is worth trying as a prophylactic measure for in-contact animals.

12. Fowl Pest. Prepared from infected discharges and used as a prophylactic given in drinking water.

13. Foot-Rot. Prepared by trituration of affected material and used as a prophylactic measure. It could also influence treatment by aiding the action of other remedies.

14. Hepatitis.   Prepared from the blood of an infected animal. It is the basis of the oral vaccine used for prevention of canine hepatitis. Can also be combined with selected remedies for treatment of actual cases.

15. Leptospirosis.   Prepared from infected urine after dilution in alcohol. Used in the same way as Hepatitis.

16. Marek's Disease.   Prepared from infected lymphoid tissue and used as a prophylactic in affected flocks.

17. Mastitis.   Various nosodes exist for the control of mastitis, e.g. those based on various species of streptococci, staphylococci, E coli and pasteurella organism, besides others. They are used in alternation on a herd basis.

18. Mucosal Disease.   Prepared from infected bowel lining and discharges. It has given encouraging results in treatment along with selected remedies.

19. Parvovirus.   Prepared from infected bowel discharges and blood. It has given good results as a prophylactic measure and is safe for all ages including the pregnant bitch.

20. Swine Dysentery.   Prepared from infected mesenteric lymph glands. It has given encouraging results in treatment along with selected remedies. It should also provide protection used as an oral vaccine.

21. Husk.   Prepared from a suspension of bronchial exudate containing the causative worms, and after trituration, dissolved in alcohol. This nosode has given good results as a prophylactic measure.

22. Scrapie.   This nosode has been prepared from brain tissue from an affected ewe. To date we have no record of its use but it should be worth trying as a prophylactic measure in affected flocks.

A Clinical Repertory

Abdomen, (distended). Abies Canadensis. Absinthum. Aesculus Glabra. Alfalfa. Allium Cepa. Aloe Socotrina. Ammonium Carbonicum. Ammonium Causticum. Anacardium Orientale. Antimonium Crudum.

Abortion. Aletris Farinosa. Caulophyllum. Cimicifuga Racemosa. Crocus Sativus. Helonias Dioica. Murex Purpurea. Pyrogenium. Sabina. Secale Cornutum. Trillium Pendulum, Ustillago Maydis. Viburnum Opulis.

Abscess. Arsenicum Album. Calcarea Sulphurica. Hepar Sulphuris. Hippozaeninum. Gunpowder. Mercurius Solubilis. Silicea. Tarentula Cubensis.

Acetonaemia. Carduus Marianus. Eucalyptus. Flor de Piedra. Lycopodium Clavatum.

Actinobacillosis. Alumen. Calcarea Fluorica. Ferrum Metallicum, Kali Iodatum. Mercurius Iodatus Flavus. Mercurius Iodatus Rubrum. Silicea.

Actinomycosis. Calcarea Fluorica. Fluoricum Acidum. Hecla Lava. Kali Iodatum.

Agalactia. Agnus Castus. Alfalfa (low potency). Fragaria Vesca. Galega Officinalis. Urtica Urens. Ustillago Maydis.

Albuminuria. Ammonium Benzoicum. Cubeba. Lithium Carbonicum. Ocimum Canum. Uranium Nitricum.

Alopecia. Arsenicum Album. Bacillinum. Lycopodium Clavatum. Sepia. Thallium Acetas. Thyroidinum. Ustillago Maydis.

Anaemia. Argentum Nitricum. Arsenicum Album. Calcarea Phosphorica. China Officinalis, Ferrum Metallicum. Manganum Acetas. Natrum Carbonicum. Natrum Muriaticum. Silicea. Trinitrotoluene. Zincum Metallicum.

Anaesthetics, (antidote to). Aceticum Acidum. Arnica Montana.

Anal adenoma. Aesculus Glabra. Nitricum Acidum. Stilboestrol.

Anal glands, (abscess of). Calcarea Sulphurica. Hepar Sulphuris. Silicea.

Anaphylaxis. Aconitum Napellus. Arnica Montana.

Aphthae. Antimonium Crudum. Antimonium Tartaricum. Borax. Mercurius Corrosivus. Muriaticum Acidum. Sulphuricum Acidum.

Appetite, (depraved) Alumina. Calcarea Carbonica.

Appetite, (lost) Nux Vomica.

Arthritis. Abrotanum. Actaea Spicata. Argentum Metallicum. Caulophyllum. Cimicifuga Racemosa. Colchicum Autumnale. Hecla Lava. Lithium Carbonicum. Nux Moschata. Radium. Rhamnus Catharticus. Rhus Toxicodendron. Ruta Graveolens. Salicylicum Acidum.

Ascites. Apis Mellifica. Apocynum Cannabinum. Cannabis Sativa. Digitalis Purpurea. Liatris Spicata. Lycopus Virginica. Strophanthus.

Atrophic Rhinitis. Fluoricum Acidum. Hecla Lava. Kali Bichromicum. Lemna Minor. Mercurius Corrosivus.

Azoturia. Berberis Vulgaris. Curare.

Balanitis. Cannabis Sativa. Mercurius Solubilis. Thuja Occidentalis.

Biliousness. Berberis Vulgaris. Lycopodium Clavatum. Nux Vomica. Sulphur.

Bites. Hypericum Perforatum. Lachesis Muta. Ledum Palustre (punctured).

Blepharitis. Aconitum Napellus. Agaricus Muscarius. Alumina. Antimonium Crudum. Apis Mellifica. Staphisagria.

Bloat. Colchicum Autumnale. Eucalyptus. Lycopodium Clavatum. Magnesium Phosphoricum. Sulphur. Terebinthinae.

Boils. Anthracinum. Gunpowder. Hepar Sulphuris. Lachesis Muta. Silicea. Tarentula Cubensis.

Bone, (injuries to) Ruta Graveolens. Symphytum.
  (exostoses of) Calcarea Carbonica. Calcarea Fluorica. Hecla Lava. Kali Bichromicum. Angustura Vera.

Bowel Oedema. Apis Mellifica. Aconitum Napellus.

Bronchitis. Ammonium Carbonicum. Ammonium Causticum. Arsenicum Album. Arsenicum Iodatum. Beryllium. Antimonium Tartaricum. Carbo Vegetabilis. Causticum. Hepar Sulphuris. Kali Bichromicum. Kali Nitricum.

Broncho-pneumonia. Antimonium Tartaricum. Baryta Carbonica. Kali Bichromicum. Kali Sulphuricum.

Bruises. Arnica Montana. Bellis Perennis. Hamamelis Virginica. Ruta Graveolens.

Burns. Cantharis Vesicatoria. Hamamelis Virginica. Urtica Urens.

Bursitis. Apis Mellifica. Hepar Sulphuris. Iodium. Ruta Graveolens.

Calf Diphtheria. Kreosotum. Lac Caninum. Mercurius Cyanatus. Mercurius Iodatus Flavus. Mercurius Iodatus Rubrum.

Canine Distemper. Aconitum Napellus. Arsenicum Album. Baptisia Tinctoria. Cicuta Virosa. Conium Maculatum. Curare. Distemperinum. Eupatorium Perfoliatum. Lycopodium Clavatum. Natrum Arsenicum. Strychninum.

Carbuncle. Anthracinum. Arsenicum Album. Lachesis Muta. Silicea. Tarentula Cubensis.

Cataract. Calcarea Carbonica. Calcarea Fluorica. Cannabis Sativa. Natrum Muriaticum. Phosphorus. Santoninum. Silicea.

Cat Enteritis, (Panleucopenia).   Arsenicum Album. Mercurius Corrosivus. Nitricum Acidum.

Cat Influenza.   Aconitum Napellus. Allium Cepa. Ammonium Muriaticum. Arsenicum Album. Euphrasia. Eupatorium Perfoliatum. Hydrastis Canadensis. Lemna Minor. Mercurius Corrosivus. Pulsatilla Nigrans. Teucrium Marum.

Cellulitis. Boracicum Acidum. Hepar Sulphuris. Kali Bichromicum. Lachesis Muta. Manganum Aceticum. Natrum Arsenicum. Rhus Toxicodendron. Secale Cornitum. Silicea.

Cerebro Cortical Necrosis. Absinthum. Agaricus Muscarius. Cicuta Virosa. Helleborus Niger. Oxytropis. Stramonium. Sulfonal. Zincum Metallicum.

Chorea. Absinthum. Agaricus Muscarius. Caslcarea Phosphorica. Cimicifuga Racemosa. Cicuta Virosa. Conium Maculatum. Hyoscyamus Niger. Ignatia Amara. Mygale Lasidora.

Coccidiosis. Allium Sativa. Ipecacuanha. Mercurius Corrosivus. Sycotic Co.

Colic (Flatulent) Aconitum Napellus. Absinthum. Acidum Hydrocyanicum. Ammonium Carbonicum. Ammonium Causticum. Carbo Vegetabilis. Colchicum Autumnale. Evonymus Europea. Euphorbium. Veratrum Album. Zingiber.

Colic, (Spasmodic).   Colocynthis. Dulcamara. Nux Vomica.

Colitis. Allium Sativa. Colchicum Autumnale. Mercurius Dulcis. Nitricum Acidum. Sycotic Co.

Conjunctivitis. Aesculus Hippocastanum. Alumina. Antimonium Crudum. Argentum Nitricum. Boracicum Acidum. Euphrasia. Kali Bichromicum. Ledum Palustre. Mercurius Solubilis.

Constipation. Aesculus Hippocastanum. Aloe Socotrina. Causticum. Gelsemium Sempervirens. Lycopodium Clavatum. Nux Vomica. Opium.

Convulsions. Absinthum. Agaricus Muscarius. Belladonna. Benzenum. Chamomilla. Cocculus. Helleborus Niger. Physostigma. Plumbum Metallicum. Stramonium. Zincum Metallicum.

Cornea, (Opacity of)   Calcarea Fluorica. Cannabis Sativa.

Cornea, (Ulceration of). Euphrasia. Kali Bichromicum. Ledum Palustre. Natrum Muriaticum.

Corns. Calcarea Carbonica. Hepar Sulphuris. Kreosotum.

Coryza. Ailanthus Glandiosa. Allium Cepa. Arsenicum Album. Bromium. Iodum. Kali Iodatum. Sulphuricum Acidum. Sulphur Iodatum.

Cough. Aesculus Hippocastanum. Antimonium Tartaricum. Ammonium Carbonicum. Ammonium Causticum. Bromium. Beryllium. Bryonia Alba. Causticum. Drosera Rotundifolia. Coccus Cacti. Hepar Sulphuris. Kali Nitricum. Ipecacuanha. Kreosotum. Lavrocerasus. Lycopodium Clavatum. Phosphorus. Pulsatilla Nigrans. Rumex Crispus. Scilla Maritima. Spongia Tosta.

Cow Pox. Antimonium Crudum. Malandrinum. Variolinum.

Cystitis. Berberis Vulgaris. Cannabis Sativa. Cantharis Vesicotoria. Causticum. Coccus Cacti. Copaiva. Cubeba. Eupatorium Purpurea. Equisetum. Ferrum Picricum. Juniperis. Lithium Carbonicum. Helonias Diocia. Populus Tremuloides. Staphisagria. Terebinthinae. Thlaspi Bursa. Triticum Pendulum. Urea. Uva Ursi. Santoninum.

Cysts, (Interdigital) Baryta Carbonica. Calcarea Fluorica. Crotalus Horridus. Graphites. Hepar Sulphuris. Phosphoricum Acidum. Secale Cornutum. Silicea. Staphisagria. Stigmata Maydis.

Dentition. Aethusa Cynapium. Calcarea Carbonica. Calcarea Phosphorica. Chamomilla. Rheum.

Diabetes. Iris Versicolor. Baryta Muriaticum. Magnesium Phosphoricum. Natrum Sulphuricum. Phaseolus. Syzygium. Uranium Nitricum. Pancreatin.

Diabetes Insipidus. Aceticum Acidum. Alfalfa. Ammonium Carbonicum. Apocynum Cannabinum. A.C.T.H. Calcarea Phosphorica. Helonias Dioica. Kali Nitricum. Phosphoricum Acidum. Uranium Nitricum. Hydrangea.

Diarrhoea. Antimonium Crudum. Arsenicum Album. Benzoicum Acidum. China Officinalis. Colchicum Autumnale. Colocynthis. Croton Tiglium. Dulcamara. Elaterium. Ferrum Metallicum. Ipecacuanha. Iris Versicolor. Jalapa. Kali Chloricum. Mercurius Corrosivus. Natrum Carbonica. Natrum Sulphuricum. Physostigma. Podophyllum. Rheum.

Digestion, (Weak) Carbo Vegetabilis. Coffea Cruda. Lycopodium Clavatum. Nux Vomica. Zingiber.

Disc, (Displaced) Hypericum Perforatum. Ruta Graveolens.

Dropsy. Apis Mellifica. Arsenicum Album. Arsenicum Iodatum. Adonis Vernalis. Colchicum Autumnale. Convallaria. Digitalis. Liatris Spicata. Strophanthus.

Dysentery. Aloe Socotrina. Cantharis Vesicotoria. Colchicum Autumnale. Crotalus Horridus. Ipecacuanha. Kali Muriaticum. Leptandra. Mercurius Corrosivus. Nitricum Acidum. Rhus Toxicodendron. Sycotic Co.

Ear Canker. Arsenicum Album. Arsenicum Iodatum. Capsicum. Elaps Corallinus. Fluoricum Acidum. Hepar Sulphuris. Malandrinum. Mercurius Corrosivus. Mercurius Dulcis. Mercurius Solubilis. Natrum Salicylicum. Psorinum. Rhus Toxicodendron. Scrophularia Nodosa. Tellurium.

Ears, (Discharge from) Borax. Hepar Sulphuris. Malandrinum. Mercurius Solubilis. Tellurium.

Eclampsia. Belladonna. Calcarea Phosphorica. Lac Caninum.

Eczema. Alumina. Anagallis Arvensis. Antimonium Crudum. Arsenicum Album. Arsenicum Iodatum. Bacillinum. Boracicum Acidum. Bovista. Bromium. Cantharis Vesicotoria. Copaiva. Croton Tiglium. Euphorbium. Graphites. Hepar Sulphuris. Iodium. Juglans Regia. Kali Arsenicum. Kali Sulphuricum. Lithium Carbonicum. Mercurius Corrosivus. Mezereum. Natrum Muriaticum. Oleander. Petroleum. Psorinum. Rhus Toxicodendron. Rhus Venenata. Salicylicum Acidum. Selenium. Sepia. Sulphur. Sulphur Iodatum. Tellurium. Urtica Urens. Vinca Minor.

Emphysema. Ammonium Carbonicum. Beryllium. Ledum Palustre. Lobelia Inflata.

Encephalitis. Belladonna. Ferrum Phosphoricum. Hyoscyamus Niger. Magnesium Phosphoricum.

Epistaxis. Aconitum Napellus. Bryonia Alba. Carbo Vegetabilis. Crotalus Horridus. Ferrum Picricum. Ferrum Phosphoricum. Ficus Religiosa. Hamamelis Virginica. Millefolium. Phosphorus. Vipera.

Excitability. Coffea Cruda. Tarentula Hispanica.

Eyes, (Injuries to) Ledum Palustre. Symphytum.

False Pregnancy. Chamomilla. Helonias Dioica. Lac Caninum. Pulsatilla.

Fear. Aconitum Napellus. Argentum Nitricum. Phosphorus. Stramonium. Hydrophorinum.

Fever. Aconitum Napellus. Aceticum Acidum. Arsenicum Album. Baptisia Tinctoria. Belladonna. Echinacea. Pyrogenium. Sulphur.

Fistula. Causicum. Calcarea Sulphurica. Fluoricum Acidum. Silicea.

Fistulous Withers. Brucella Abortus. Hepar Sulphuris. Silicea.

Fits. (See Convulsions)

Fog Fever. Adonis Vernalis. Ammonium Causticum. Ammonium Muriaticum. Antimonium Tartaricum. Apis Mellifica. Beryllium. Fluoricum Acidum. Kali Iodatum.

Foot-Rot. Kreosotum. Hepar Sulphuris. Silicea.

Foul in Foot. Hepar Sulphuris. Kreosotum. Silicea. Malandrinum.

Fowl Paralysis. Conium Maculatum. Lathyrus Sativus.

Gastritis. Abies Canadensis. Abies Nigra. Arsenicum Album. Chamomilla. Ferrum Metallicum. Ferrum Phosphoricum. Lobelia Inflata. Phosphorus.

Gastro-Enteritis. Arsenicum Album. Bismuthum. Iris Versicolor. Kali Nitricum. Podophyllum. Veratrum Album.

Glands, (enlarged) Alumen. Baryta Carbonica. Bromium. Calcarea Carbonica. Hepar Sulphuris. Kali Iodatum. Phytolacca Decandra.

Glaucoma. Osmium. Phosphorus.

Grass Sickness. Plumbum Metallicum. Gelsemium Sempervirens. Lathyrus Sativa. Opium.

Gravel. Hydrangea. Thlaspi Bursa.

Grease. Kali Bichromicum. Malandrinum. Variolinum.

Haematoma. Arnica Montana. Crotalus Horridus. Melilotus.

Haematuria. Berberis Vulgaris. Erigeron. Ficus Religiosa. Millefolium. Phosphorus. Terebinthinae.

Haemoglobinuria. Berberis Vulgaris. Coccus Cacti. Hamamelis Virginica. Santoninum.

Haemoptysis. Aconitum Napellus. Ferrum Phosphoricum. Hamamelis Virginica. Phosphorus.

Haemorrhage, (Remedies in General) Arnica Montana. Bothrops Lanceolatus. Ceanothus. China Officinalis. Crocus Sativa. Crotalus Horridus. Erigeron. Hamamelis Virginica. Ferrum Phosphoricum. Ficus Religiosa. Ipecacuanha. Melilotus. Millefolium. Muriaticum Acidum. Sabina. Secale Cornutum. Trillium Pendulum.

Heart, (Remedies in General) Adonis Vernalis. Arnica Montana. Cactus Grandiflorus. Convallaria Majus. Crataegus. Digitalis. Iberis. Kalmia Latifolia. Laurocerasus. Lycopus Virginica. Naja Tripudians. Phaseolus. Serum Anguillar Ichthotoxin (Eel Serum). Spartium Scoparium. Spongia Tosta. Squilla Maritima. Strophanthus.

Heat Stroke. Belladonna.

Hepatitis. Berberis Vulgaris. Carduus Marianus. Chelidonium Majus, Crotalus Horridus. Elaps Corallinus. Kali Muriaticum. Leptandra. Manganum Aceticum. Lycopodium Clavatum. Mercurius Dulcis. Mercurius Iodatus Flavus. Mercurius Iodatus Rubrum. Mercurius Solubilis. Natrum Sulphuricum. Ptelea.

Herpes. Borax. Natrum Muriaticum. Nitricum Acidum. Ranunculus Bulbosus. Rhus Toxicodendron.

Hodgkins Disease. Benzenum. Calcarea Fluorica. Cistus Canadensis. Kali Muriaticum. Phytolacca Decandra.

Hypomagnesaemia. Agaricus Muscarius. Belladonna. Gelsemium. Hyoscyamus Niger. Mygale Lasidora. Mygale Lasidora. Magnesium Phosphoricum. Stramonium.

Hysteria Agaricus Muscarius. Belladonna. Benzoicum Acidum. Hyosyamus Niger. Ignatia Amara. Platina. Scutellaria. Stramonium. Tarentula Hispanica.

Iliac Thrombosis. Bothrops Lanceolatus. Crotalus Horridus. Lachesis Muta. Secale Cornutum. Vipera.

Incontinence. Conium Maculatum. Lobelia Inflata. Causticum.

Indigestion. Anacardium Orientale. Carbo Vegetabilis. Nux Vomica.

Indurations. Alumen. Calcarea Fluorica. Condurango.

Infertility, (Remedies in General) Calcarea Phosphorica. Caulophyllum. Lilium Tigrinum. Manganum Aceticum. Murex Purpurea. Palladium. Platina. Pulsatilla Nigrans. Sepia.

Influenza. Baptisia Tinctora. Curare. Eupatorium Perfoliatum. Gelsemium Sempervirens. Lathyrus. Lobelia Inflata.

Injuries. Arnica Montana. Bellis Perennis. Hypericum Perforatum. Ledum Palustre. Symphytum.

Insect Bites. Cantharis Vesicotoria. Ledum Palustre.

Jaundice. Berberis Vulgaris. Carduus Marianus. Chelidonium Majus. China Officinalis. Crotalus Horridus. Hydrastis Canadensis. Iris Versicolor. Juglans Regia. Lachesis Muta. Leptandra. Mercurius Dulcis. Myrica. Natrum Sulphuricum. Podophyllum. Senecio Aureus. Thyroidenum. Vipera.

Joints, (Remedies in General) Apis Mellifica. Bryonia Alba. Caulophyllum. Causticum. Colchicum Autumnale. Kali Iodatum. Ledum Palustre. Rhus Toxicodendron.

Joint-Ill. Apis Mellifica. Hepar Sulphuris. Streptococcus.

Keratitis. Mercurius Corrosivus. Kali Bichromicum. Sanguinaria Canadensis. Silicea.

Kidneys, (Remedies in General). Adonis Vernalis. Ammonium Benzoicum. Antimonium Crudum. Apis Mellifica. Apocynum Cannabinum. Benzoicum Acidum. Cannabis Sativa. Cantharis Vesicotoria. Chimaphilla Umbellata. Dulcamara. Euonymus Europea. Eupatorium Purpureum. Equisetum. Erigeron. Fluoricum Acidum. Hepar Sulphuris. Juniperis. Kali Carbonicum. Kali Chloricum. Lithium Carbonicum. Magnesium Sulphuricum. Mercurius Corrosivus. Mercurius Cyanatus. Mercurius Solubilis. Natrum Muriaticum. Ocimum Canum. Phosphorus. Picricum Acidum. Populus Tremuloides. Plumbum Metallicum. Prunus Spinosa. Radium. Sambucus Niger. Selenium. Senecio Aureus. Solidago Virga. Spartium Scoparus. Squilla Maritima. Terebinthinae. Triticum. Urea. Urtica Urens.

Lactation, (Deficient).   See Agalactia

Lactation, (Excessive). Alfalfa (high potency). Lac Caninum. Uranium Nitricum. Ustillago Maydis.

Laminitis.   Aconitum Napellus. Belladonna. Calcarea Fluorica.

Laryngitis.   Allium Cepa. Antimonium Tartaricum. Apis Mellifica. Arsenicum Iodatum. Carbo Vegetabilis. Causticum. Drosera Rotundifolia. Hepar Sulphuris. Iodium. Kali Iodatum. Lachesis Muta. Osmium. Spongia Tosta.

Leptospirosis.   Crotalus Horridus.   Lycopodium.   Chelidonium Majus. Berberis Vulgaris.

Liver, (Remedies in General)   Abies Canadensis. Absinthum. Aesculus Hippocastanum. Aloe Socotrina. Ammonium Muriaticum. Berberis Vulgaris. Carduus Marianus. Chelidonium Majus. Euonymus Europea. Flor De Piedra. Iris Versicolor. Juglans Regia. Kali Carbonicum. Leptandra. Lycopodium Clavatum. Magnesium Muriaticum. Mercurius Dulcis. Myrica. Natrum Sulphuricum. Phosphorus. Podophyllum. Ptelea. Plumbum Metallicum. Senecio Aureus. Sulphur. Uranium Nitricum. Vipera.

Louping-Ill.   Agaricus Muscarius. Oxytropis.

Lungs, (Congestion of)   Antimonium Tartaricum. Ammonium Carbonicum. Ammonium Causticum. Apis Mellifica. Berberis Vulgaris. Bothrops Lanceolatus. Carbo Vegetabilis. Crocus Sativus. Drosera Rotundifolia. Ferrum Phosphoricum. Hydrastus Canadensis. Kali Iodatum. Kali Muriaticum. Phosphorus. Sanguinaria. Veratrum Viride.

Lymphadenitis.   Alumen. Bromium. Calcarea Fluorica. Cistus Canadensis. Conium Maculatum. Hepar Sulphuris. Kali Muriaticum. Mercurius Iodatus Flavus. Mercurius Iodatus Rubrum. Mercurius Solubilis. Phytolacca Decandra. Rumex Crispus. Scrophularia Nodosa. Spongia Tosta. Trifolium Pratense. Vipera.

Lymphangitis.   Aceticum Acidum. Kali Bichromicum. Lachesis Muta. Malandrinum. Muriaticum Acidum. Elaps Corallinus. Tarentula Cubensis.

Mammary Glands, (Remedies in General).   Aceticum Acidum. Alumen. Bufo. Calcarea Fluorica. Carbo Animalis. Conium Maculatum. Hepar Sulphuris. Hydrastis Canadensis. Lac Caninum. Lachesis Muta. Phytolacca Decandra. Scrophularia Nodosa. Silicea. Thyroidenum.

Mastitis.   Belladonna, Bryonia Alba. Calcarea Fluorica. Cistus Canadensis. Hepar Sulphuris. Phosphorus. Phytolacca Decandra. Pulsatilla Nigrans.

Meningitis.   Agaricus Muscarius. Belladonna. Cicuta Virosa. Ferrum Phosphoricum.

Metritis. Aconitum Napellus. Aletris Farinosa. Baptisia Tinctora. Caulophyllum. Echinacea. Helonias Dioica. Hydrastis Canadensis. Cantharis Vesicotoria. Crotalus Horridus. Lilium Tigrinum. Pulsatilla Nigrans. Pyrogenium. Sabina. Secale Cornutum. Sepia.

Metrorrhagia. Bovista. Bufo. Erigeron. Ficus Religiosa. Ipecacuanha. Sabina. Secale Cornutum. Ustillago Maydis. Alestris Farinosa.

Milk, (Blood in). Bufo. Phosphorus. Ipecacuanha.

Milk Fever, (Remedies for Supportive Treatment). Agaricus Muscarius. Belladonna. Calcarea Carbonica. Calcarea Phosphorica. Stramonium.

Mouth, (Ulceration of). Aceticum Acidum. Borax. Kali Chloricum. Mercurius Cyanatus. Mercurius Solubilis. Muriaticum Acidum.

Mucosal Disease. Allium Sativa. Ammonium Causticum. Borax. Hydrastis Canadensis. Kali Sulphuricum. Magnesium Carbonicum. Nitricum Acidum. Sycotic Co. Trillium Pendulum.

Nails, (Brittle). Calcarea Phosphorica. Secale Cornutum. Silicea.

Navicular Disease. Apis Mellifica. Crotalus Horridus. Rhus Toxicodendron. Ruta Graveolens. Vipera.

Nephritis. (See Kidney).

Nervousness. Argentum Nitricum. Borax. Bufo. Gelsemium Sempervirnes. Magnesium Carbonicum. Magnesium Phosphoricum. Mygale Lasidora. Phosphorus. Tarentula Hispanica.

New Forest Disease. Cannabis Sativa. Kali Iodatum. Silicea.

Oedema. Antipyrene. Apis Mellifica. Digitalis. Liatris Spicata. Strophanthus. Urtica Urens.

Ophthalmia. Argentum Nitricum. Chelidonium Majus. Hepar Sulphuris. Ruta Graveolens.

Orchitis. Benzenum. Cannabis Sativa. Phytolacca Decandra. Rhododendron. Spongia Tosta. Ustillago Maydis.

Osteomalacia. Calcarea Carbonica. Calcarea Phosphorica.

Otorrhoea. Hepar Sulphuris. Malandrinum. Mercurius Corrosivus. Psorinum.

Ovaritis. Cimicifuga Racemosa. Eupatorium Purpureum. Palladium. Platina. Pulsatilla Nigrans. Vespa.

Ovary, (Remedies in General). Iodium. Lilium Tigrinum. Murex Purpurea. Palladium Platina. Pulsatilla Nigrans. Vespa.

Pancreatitis. Baryta Muriaticum. Boracicum Acidum. Flor De Piedra. Iris Versicolor. Kali Iodatum. Mercurius Solubilis. Pancreatin.

Panleucopenia. (See Cat Enteritis)

Papilloma. Thuja

Paraplegia. Bothrops Lanceolatus. Causticum. Conium Maculatum. Curare. Hypericum Perforatum. Lathyrus Sativa. Plumbum Metallicum.

Parotitis. Kali Muriaticum. Lachesis Muta. Mercurius Iodatus Flavus. Mercurius Iodatus Rubrum. Parotidinum. Phytolacca Decandra. Pilocarpus. Pulsatilla Nigrans.

Parvovirus Disease. Arsenicum Album. Iris Versicolor. Phosphorus.

Pedal Ostitis. Calcarea Fluorica. Ruta Graveolens. Hecla Lava.

Periodic Ophthalmia. Natrum Muriaticum. Cannabis Sativa.

Peritonitis. Aconitum Napellus. Hepar Sulphuris. Palladium. Arsenicum Album. Cantharis Vesicotoria. Rhus Toxicodendron.

Pharyngitis. Aesculus Hippocastanum. Capsicum. Ferrum Phosphoricum. Kali Chloricum. Lac Caninum. Lachesis Muta. Mercurius Cyanatus. Mercurius Iodatus Flavus. Mercurius Iodatus Rubrum. Natrum Arsenicum. Phytolacca Decandra. Salicylicum Acidum. Vinca Minor.

Placenta, (Retained). Caulophyllum. Pulsatilla Nigrans. Sabina. Secale Cornutum. Pyrogenium. Agnus Castus.

Pleurisy. Aconitum Napellus. Apis Mellifica. Bryonia Alba. Hepar Sulphuris. Phaseolus. Rhus Toxicodendron.

Pneumonia. Aconitum Napellus. Ammonium Carbonicum. Ammonium Causticum. Antimonium Tartaricum. Arsenicum Iodatum. Beryllium. Bryonia Alba. Drosera Rotundiflora. Kali Iodatum. Kreosotum. Lycopodium Clavatum. Phosphorus.

Poll Evil. Hepar Sulphuris. Silicea. Brucella Abortus.

Polyuria. Abies Canadensis. Absinthum. Aceticum Acidum. Aesculus Hippocastanum. Aethusa Cynapium. Agaricus Muscarius. Allium Cepa. Antimonium Crudum. Bismuthum. Boracicum Acidum. Apocynum Cannabinum. Uranium Nitricum.

Pregnancy Toxaemia. Lycopodium Clavatum. Phosphorus. Calcarea Phosphorica.

Prostate, (Enlarged). Chimaphilla Umbellata. Conium Maculatum. Eupatorium Purpurea. Ferrum Picricum. Kali Iodatum. Phytolacca Decandra. Picricum Acidum. Populus Tremuloides. Solidago Virga. Stigmata Maydis. Triticum. Hydrangea.

Puerperal Fever. Crotalus Horridus. Echinacea. Lachesis Muta. Terebinthinae.

Purpura Haemorrhagica. Crotalus Horridus. Haemamelis Virginica. Phosphorus. Sulphuricum Acidum.

Pyelitis. Hepar Sulphuris. E. Coli. Juniperis. Kali Bichromicum. Uva Ursi.

Pyelonephritis. Eucalyptus. Hepar Sulphuris. E. Coli.

Pyometra. Caulophyllum. Cimicifuga Racemosa. Copaiva. Echinacea. Hydrastis Canadensis. Kali Bichromicum. Lilium Tigrinum. Pulsatilla Nigrans. Pyrogenium. Sabina. Secale Cornutum. Sepia.

Quittor. Silicea. Calcarea Sulphurica.

Ranula. Ammonium Benzoicum.
Retinal Atrophy. Phosphorus.
Rhinitis. Allium Cepa. Hydrastis Canadensis. Fluoricum Acidum. Kali Bichromicum. Lemna Minor. Mercurius Corrosivus.
Rhino-Pneumonitis. Arsenicum Iodatum. Beryllium. Hippozaeninum. Phosphorus.
Rickets. Calcarea Carbonica. Calcarea Phosphorica.
Ringbone. Calcarea Carbonica. Hecla Lava. Ruta Graveolens.
Ringwomb. Caulophyllum. Veratrum Viride.
Ringworm. Bacillinum. Arsenicum Album. Dulcamara. Kali Sulphuricum. Selenium. Sepia. Tellurium.
Roaring, (In Horses). Lathyrus Sativa. Gelsemium Sempervirens.
Rodent Ulcer. Alumen. Capsicum. Cistus Canadensis. Conium Maculatum. Muriaticum Acidum. Nitricum Acidum.

Salivation, (Excessive). Bromium. Eserine. Mercurius Solubilis. Nitricum Acidum. Iodium. Pilocarpus. Ptelea. Trifolium Pratense.
Sandcrack. Silicea. Calcarea Fluorica.
Satyriasis. Tarentula Hispanica. Ustillago Maydis. Yohimbinum.
Sebaceous Cysts. Calcarea Fluorica. Kali Bromatum.
Septicaemia. Baptisia Tinctora. Bufo. Echinacea. Elaps Corallinus. Crotalus Horridus. Kreosotum. Lachesis Muta. Tarentula Cubensis. Veratrum Viride. Zincum Metallicum.
Sesamoiditis. Calcarea Fluorica. Hecla Lava. Ruta Graveolens.
Shock. Aconitum Napellus. Arnica Montagu. Camphora. Carbo Vegetabilis. Opium.
Sinus (and Fistula) Calcarea Sulphurica. Hepar Sulphuris. Silicea.
Sinusitis. Hepar Sulphuris. Kali Bichromium. Natrum Muriaticum.
Spavin. Aesculus Hippocastanum. Angustura Vera. Apis Mellifica. Calcarea Carbonica. Calcarea Fluorica. Hecla Lava.
Spine, (Injuries to). Hypericum Perforatum. Ruta Graveolens.
Splenitis. Ceanothus. Eucalyptus.
Splint. Calcarea Fluorica. Hecla Lava. Ruta Graveolens.
Sprains. Arnica Montana. Bellis Perennis. Rhus Toxicodendron. Ruta Graveolens.
Stings. Apis Mellifica. Echinacea. Ledum Palustre. Vespa.
Stomatitis. Kali Chloricum. Borax. Mercurius Solubilis. Muriaticum Acidum. Salicylicum Acidum. Sulphuricum Acidum. Trifolium Pratense.
Strangles. Hepar Sulphuris. Silicea. Staphylococcus Aureus.

Stuttgart's Disease. Alumina. Arsenicum Iodatum. Arsenicum Album. Baptisia Tinctoria. Mercurius Cyanatus. Mercurius Solubilis. Pyrogenium.

Sun (Effects of) Aconitum Napellus. Belladonna. Glonoine.

Sweet Itch. Arsenicum Album. Kali Arsenicum. Malandrinum. Variolinum.

Swine Dysentery. Arsenicum Album. Sycotic Co. Trillium Pendulum.

Swine Erysipelas. Belladonna. Morbillinum.

Synovitis. Apis Mellifica. Bryonia Alba. Eupatorium Perfoliatum. Iodium.

Teething. Chamomilla.

Tendons, (Contracted). Causticum.

Tendons, (Sprained). Arnica Montana. Hypericum Perforatum. Rhus Toxicodendron. Ruta Graveolens.

Thoroughpin. Apis Mellifica. Bryonia Alba. Iodium.

Throat, (Remedies in General). Capsicum. Causticum. Kali Bichromicum. Mercurius Iodatus Flavus. Mercurius Iodatus Rubrum. Mercurius Cyanatus. Phytolacca Decandra.

Thyroid Gland. Flor De Piedra. Iodium. Kali Iodatum. Spongia Tosta.

Tongue, (Remedies in General). Alumen. Borax. Bryonia Alba. Kali Chloricum. Mercurius Solubilis.

Tonsillitis. Baryta Carbonica. Bromium. Hepar Sulphuris. Lac Caninum.

Torticollis. Aesculus Glabra. Cicuta Virosa.

Toxaemia. Echinacea. Pyrogenium. Vanadium.

Travel Sickness. Cocculus Indicus.

Tympany. (See Bloat).

Urethritis. Coccus Cacti. Copaiva. Cubeba. Juniperis. Thlaspi Bursa.

Urine, (Blood in). (See Haematuria).

Urine, (Discoloured). (Remedies in General). Absinthum. Aconitum Napellus. Aesculus Hippocastanum. Aethusa Cynapium. Allium Cepa. Ammonium Benzoicum. Ammonium Muriaticum. Antimonium Crudum. Benzoicum Acidum. Carbolicum Acidum. Colchicum Autumnale. Lycopodium Clavatum. Magnesium Sulphuricum. Myrica.

Urine, (Sediment in). Kali Chloricum. Lycopodium Clavatum. Phosphoricum Acidum.

Urine, (Slimy). Copaiva. Ocimum Canum.

Urticaria. Apis Mellifica. Ledum Palustre. Rhus Toxicodendron. Urtica Urens.

Uterus, (Bleeding from). (See Metrorrhagia).
Uterus, (Inflammation of). (See Metritis).
Umbilicus, (Patent). Abrotanum. Nux Vomica.

Vesicular stomatitis. Antimonium Crudum.
Vomiting, (Remedies in General). Abies Canadensis. Abies Nigra. Aethusa Cynapium. Alumina. Antimonium Tartaricum. Apomorphinum. Arsenicum Album. Ipecacuanha. Iris Versicolor. Phosphorus.

Warts. Calcarea Carbonica. Causticum. Dulcamara. Ferrum Picricum. Nitricum Acidum. Selenium. Thuja Occidentalis.
White Scour, (in Calves). Aethus Cynapium. Allium Sativa. Arsenicum Album. Camphora. China Officinalis. Croton Tiglium. E. Coli. Ipecacuanha. Magnesium Carbonicum. Veratrum Album. Angustura Vera.
Windgalls. Apis Mellifica. Eupatorium Perfoliatum.
Worms, (Round). Abrotanum. Cina Maritima. Ferrum Metallicum. Santoninum. Teucrium Marum.
Worms, (Tape). Filix Mas. Granatum. Kousso.
Wounds, (Open). Crotalus Horridus. Hypericum Perforatum. Calendula Officinalis.
Wounds, (Punctured or Stab). Ledum Palustre. Hypericum Perforatum.